Essential MCQs for Medical Finals

Rema Kaur Wasan BA MBBS MA MRCP FRCR

Specialist Registrar Radiology
St Georges Hospital, London

Delilah Hassanally BSc MBBS MSc FRCS

Specialist Registrar Surgery
Old Church Hospital, Essex

Balvinder Singh Wasan BSc MBBS MRCP

Specialist Registrar Cardiology
St Mary's Hospital, London

Egerton Court
Parkgate Estate
Knutsford
Cheshire WA16 8DX

Telephone: 01565 752000

First published 1997
Reprinted 1999
Second edition 2002

ISBN 1 901198 20 0

A catalogue record for this book is available from the British Library.

Typeset by Breeze Limited, Manchester.
Printed by Bell and Bain Ltd., Glasgow.

CONTENTS

INTRODUCTION

There are many multiple choice question books for postgraduate medical examinations, and for years undergraduates preparing for finals have been forced to struggle with these as there is very little revision material specific to their needs.

The aim of this book is to provide 'real' MCQ practice examinations at the appropriate level for undergraduates sitting their final medical examinations. These questions will also benefit those sitting the PLAB examination.

This book contains three test papers designed to be similar in format, content and balance of subjects to medical finals MCQ examinations. Answers and detailed teaching notes are given for each question. The questions are as 'real' as possible; they include material that has been remembered by medical students after their medical finals examinations. There is a natural tendency to recall the harder and more confusing topics, but rather than avoiding these, we have deliberately included them and so the pass mark for each paper is probably a little less than 50%. We hope medical students will use this to their advantage; everyone will get the easy questions right, but the medical student who enters the examination having done the more difficult questions should not just pass, but pass well.

The second edition contains extra questions to cover recent developments. In addition, we have revised questions according to changes in current medical opinion and to reflect changes in examination emphasis.

Rema Wasan
Delilah Hassanally
Balvinder Wasan

MCQ EXAMINATION TECHNIQUE

Before sitting an MCQ examination, you will need to know how many questions are likely to be on the paper and how long you will be given to complete it. Thus you will be able to assess the approximate amount of time that can be spent on each question. Pacing yourself accurately during the examination to finish on time, or with time to spare, is essential.

In MCQ examinations you must read the question (both stem and items A–E) carefully. Take care not to mark the wrong boxes and think very carefully before making a mark on the answer sheet. Regard each item as being independent of every other item – each refers to a specific quantum of knowledge. The item (or the stem and the item taken together) make up a statement. You are required to indicate whether you regard this statement as 'True' or 'False'. Look only at a single statement when answering – disregard all the other statements presented in the question. They have nothing to do with the item you are concentrating on.

As you go through the questions, you can either mark your answers immediately on the answer sheet or you can mark them on the question paper and then transfer them to the answer sheet. If you adopt the second approach you must take great care not to make any errors and not to run out of time, since you will not be allowed extra time to transfer marks to the answer sheet. The answer sheet must always be marked neatly and carefully according to the instructions given. Careless marking is probably one of the commonest causes of rejection of answer sheets by the document reader.

- Do as many good quality practice papers as possible. This will help you to identify your strengths and weaknesses in time for further study. You can also use the Revision Index at the back of this book to find questions on specific topics, so that after you have done some reading you can test your knowledge.

- With the three exams provided in this book be strict with yourself and work under realistic exam conditions. You should develop an understanding of your own work rate so that you know how much time you can spend on each question.

- Read each question several times. Nobody at this vital stage in their career should be wasting marks because they misread or misunderstood the question.

- Each exam in this book contains 60 questions.

- If you have to guess the answer to a question, put a special mark next to it. You will then be able to find out if you are a good guesser. This is especially important if your examination is negatively marked, i.e. marks will be deducted for incorrect answers. It is important to know what you know as well as what you don't know.

- Use the Revision Checklist on the following pages to keep a record of the subjects you have covered and feel confident about. This will ensure that you do not miss out any key topics.

SAMPLE ANSWER SHEET

UNIVERSITY OF LONDON Management Systems Division

MULTIPLE-CHOICE EXAMINATION ANSWER SHEET

DATE ....

SURNAME ....

FIRST NAME(S) ....

Instructions: Use the HB pencil provided. To make an answer draw a single horizontal line along the dotted line **above** the appropriate letter or number. To answer 'TRUE' draw your line **above** the capital letter in the upper row. To answer 'FALSE' draw your line **above** the lower case letter in the lower row. For example:

[A] / [a] for 'TRUE'   [A] / [a] for 'FALSE'

If you change your mind and wish to cancel a completed answer, draw another line **below** the letter or number, along the dotted line. **Do not rub out.**

Candidate No.				Test No.				College No.	
0	0	0	0	e	0	0	0	0	0
1	1	1	1	I	1	1	1	1	1
2	2	2	2	P	2	2	2	2	2
3	3	3	3		3	3	3	3	3
4	4	4	4		4	4	4	4	4
5	5	5	5		5	5	5	5	5
6	6	6	6		6	6	6	6	6
7	7	7	7		7	7	7	7	7
8	8	8	8		8	8	8	8	8
9	9	9	9		9	9	9	9	9

Shown below is the correct method of completion, the correct method of cancellation/alteration and examples of various incorrect methods of completion.

CORRECT METHOD OF COMPLETION

True = [A] / [a]   False = [A] / [a]

CORRECT METHOD OF CANCELLATION/ ALTERATION

To cancel a response, draw a line below the letter. Do not rub out. Thus:

[A] / [a] or [A] / [a] = Cancelled

To alter a response, first cancel. Then draw a line above the other letter. Thus:

False = [A] / [a]   True = [A] / [a]

INCORRECT METHODS OF COMPLETION

Too faint [A]

Slanted [A]

Too low [A]

Too high [A]

Into next box [A] [B]

Too short [A] [A] [A]

Isolated cancellation [A]

DETERMINATE TYPE T

Each question number below has the boxes [A] [B] [C] [D] [E] in the upper row and [a] [b] [c] [d] [e] in the lower row.

1	13	25	37	49
2	14	26	38	50
3	15	27	39	51
4	16	28	40	52
5	17	29	41	53
6	18	30	42	54
7	19	31	43	55
8	20	32	44	56
9	21	33	45	57
10	22	34	46	58
11	23	35	47	59
12	24	36	48	60

KENRICK & JEFFERSON MP 20 3077 20M 8.95 Printers to the Computer Industry

REVISION CHECKLIST

Use this checklist to record your revision progress. Tick the subjects when you feel confident that you have covered them adequately. This will ensure that you do not forget to revise any key topics. This list is arranged in approximate order of importance. Items closest to the top of each list are most likely to come up in examinations.

CARDIOLOGY

❑ Arrhythmias
❑ Atrial fibrillation
❑ Heart block
❑ first degree, second degree
❑ complete heart block
❑ Ventricular tachycardia
❑ Ventricular fibrillation
❑ Wolff-Parkinson-White syndrome
❑ Sick sinus syndrome
❑ Electrocardiogram (ECG) components and changes in: angina; pericarditis; myocardial infarction;hypothermia; common arrhythmias
❑ JVP waveform
❑ Cardiac failure
❑ Ischaemic heart disease
❑ Angina
❑ Myocardial infarction
❑ Pericardial disease
❑ Hypertension
❑ primary
❑ secondary
❑ Valvular dysfunction, in particular aortic, mitral
Some questions about Carey-Coombs, Austin Flint and Graham Steell murmurs have appeared in past papers
❑ Endocarditis
❑ Rheumatic fever
❑ Features of HOCM
❑ Marfan's syndrome

RESPIRATORY SYSTEM

- ❑ Bronchial cancer
- ❑ Asthma
- ❑ Pleural effusion
- ❑ COAD
- ❑ Pneumonia
- ❑ Cystic fibrosis
- ❑ Lung fibrosis
- ❑ Asbestos exposure
- ❑ Sarcoid
- ❑ Haemoptysis

GASTROENTEROLOGY

- ❑ Peptic ulceration
- ❑ Dysphagia
- ❑ Jaundice
- ❑ Fat malabsorption
- ❑ Cirrhosis
- ❑ Hepatitis – drug or metabolic causes
- ❑ Crohn's disease
- ❑ Ulcerative colitis
- ❑ Hepatic encephalopathy
- ❑ Irritable bowel syndrome
- ❑ Diverticular disease
- ❑ Bowel malignancy
- ❑ Zollinger-Ellison syndrome – an uncommon condition but a common question in examinations

NEUROPATHY

- ❑ Stroke
- ❑ Spastic paraparesis
- ❑ Multiple sclerosis
- ❑ Motor neurone disease
- ❑ Parkinson's disease
- ❑ Cerebellar lesion
- ❑ Frontal lobe syndrome
- ❑ Visual field defects
- ❑ Papilloedema
- ❑ Peripheral neuropathy
- ❑ Ptosis
- ❑ Reflexes

- ❑ Plantar responses
- ❑ Epilepsy – especially clinical features of TLE and management of status epilepticus
- ❑ Dementia
- ❑ Carpal tunnel syndrome

METABOLIC MEDICINE

- ❑ Diabetes mellitus
- ❑ Thyroid dysfunction
- ❑ Lipid abnormalities
- ❑ Hirsutism
- ❑ Acromegaly
- ❑ Vitamin D deficiency
- ❑ Osteomalacia
- ❑ Rickets (rare)
- ❑ Causes of hypercalcaemia

RENAL

- ❑ Nephrotic syndrome
- ❑ Urinary tract infection
- ❑ Renal stones
- ❑ Nephritis, including glomerulonephritis
- ❑ Polyuria
- ❑ Oliguria

CONNECTIVE TISSUE DISEASE/RHEUMATOLOGY

- ❑ Systemic lupus erythematosus
- ❑ Rheumatoid arthritis
- ❑ Polymyositis and polymyalgia – especially the difference between the two
- ❑ Sarcoid
- ❑ Temporal arteritis
- ❑ Mixed connective tissue disease
- ❑ Raynaud's phenomenon

HAEMATOLOGY

- ❑ Causes of increased/decreased red cells, white cells
- ❑ Platelets

1.20 Syncope is a recognised feature of

- ❑ A pertussis
- ❑ B Menière's disease
- ❑ C hypertrophic obstructive cardiomyopathy
- ❑ D complete heart block
- ❑ E paroxysmal tachycardia

1.21 Glycosuria may be found in

- ❑ A normal patients
- ❑ B Cushing's syndrome
- ❑ C Addison's disease
- ❑ D Fanconi syndrome
- ❑ E acromegaly

1.22 Recognised causes of diarrhoea include

- ❑ A chronic pancreatitis
- ❑ B thyrotoxicosis
- ❑ C carcinoid syndrome
- ❑ D hyperparathyroidism
- ❑ E diabetes mellitus

1.23 Hypercalcaemia can occur in

- ❑ A pseudohypoparathyroidism
- ❑ B pseudopseudohypoparathyroidism
- ❑ C sarcoid
- ❑ D acute pancreatitis
- ❑ E Paget's disease

1.24 The following statements about the normal chest X-ray are correct:

- ❑ A the left hemidiaphragm is lower than the right
- ❑ B the left hilum is higher than the right
- ❑ C the trachea is slightly to the left of the midline
- ❑ D the heart appears larger on a PA film
- ❑ E the horizontal fissure is normally visible on the left

1.25 Causes of papilloedema include

- ❏ A hyperparathyroidism
- ❏ B type II respiratory failure
- ❏ C hypertension
- ❏ D benign intracranial hypertension
- ❏ E parasagittal meningioma

1.26 Cystic fibrosis

- ❏ A occurs in 1 in 20,000 live births
- ❏ B has sex-linked recessive inheritance
- ❏ C causes clubbing
- ❏ D usually leads to death in the early teens
- ❏ E causes steatorrhoea

1.27 Pulmonary embolism often produces the following:

- ❏ A pleuritic chest pain
- ❏ B tachypnoea, tachycardia and hypoxia
- ❏ C loud P2
- ❏ D ECG pattern of S1 Q3 T3
- ❏ E cardiomegaly

1.28 Dysphagia occurs with

- ❏ A iron deficiency
- ❏ B myasthenia gravis
- ❏ C Chagas disease
- ❏ D anxiety
- ❏ E pyloric stenosis

1.29 Acromegaly causes

- ❏ A glycosuria
- ❏ B blindness
- ❏ C hypertension
- ❏ D cardiomyopathy
- ❏ E hepatomegaly

1.30 The risk of osteoporosis is increased in

- ❑ A Asians
- ❑ B thyrotoxicosis
- ❑ C premature menopause
- ❑ D steroid therapy
- ❑ E heparin treatment

1.31 Ocular complications of diabetes mellitus include

- ❑ A retinitis pigmentosa
- ❑ B optic neuritis
- ❑ C new vessel formation in the retina
- ❑ D an isolated third nerve palsy
- ❑ E glaucoma

1.32 The usual biochemical features of primary hyperaldosteronism include

- ❑ A hypokalaemia
- ❑ B hypernatraemia
- ❑ C metabolic acidosis
- ❑ D increased plasma renin activity
- ❑ E hypotension

1.33 The following statements about Type I (insulin dependent) diabetes are true:

- ❑ A diabetic nephropathy affects about 4% of all subjects
- ❑ B retinopathy is less common than with Type II diabetes
- ❑ C there is an increased frequency of HLA DR3
- ❑ D nephropathy is more common than retinopathy
- ❑ E insulin dosage must be decreased when illness prevents eating and drinking

1.34 Nephrotic syndrome may be caused by

- ❑ A congenital defects
- ❑ B systemic lupus erythematosus (SLE)
- ❑ C retinal vein thrombosis
- ❑ D interstitial nephritis
- ❑ E gold

1.35 In Paget's disease

- ❑ A symptoms are proportional to the degree of skeletal involvement
- ❑ B serum calcium is usually elevated
- ❑ C plasma acid phosphatase is elevated
- ❑ D cardiac failure is a recognised complication
- ❑ E about 10% of patients develop osteosarcoma

1.36 The following enable a diagnosis of diabetes mellitus to be made:

- ❑ A random plasma glucose of 12 mmol/l
- ❑ B fasting plasma glucose of 6.8 mmol/l
- ❑ C islet cell antibodies
- ❑ D glycosuria
- ❑ E retinal new vessel formation

1.37 The following are causes of a ptosis:

- ❑ A dystrophia myotonica
- ❑ B myasthenia gravis
- ❑ C facial nerve palsy
- ❑ D damage to the parasympathetic nervous system
- ❑ E damage to the sympathetic nervous system

1.38 The following may be features of a Bell's palsy:

- ❑ A pain
- ❑ B hyperacusis
- ❑ C loss of taste in the anterior part of the tongue
- ❑ D ptosis
- ❑ E deafness

1.39 The following may be presenting features of acute myocardial infarction:

- ❑ A confusion
- ❑ B acute pulmonary oedema
- ❑ C syncope
- ❑ D diabetic hyperglycaemic states
- ❑ E fall

1.40 Cardiac causes of finger clubbing include

- ❑ A transposition of the vessels
- ❑ B maladie de Roger
- ❑ C atrial septal defect
- ❑ D rheumatic fever
- ❑ E Fallot's tetralogy

1.41 In the management of a cardiac arrest

- ❑ A DC cardioversion is seldom useful in ventricular fibrillation
- ❑ B external cardiac compression should depress the sternum 1.5–2 inches
- ❑ C hypovolaemia may be a cause of electromechanical dissociation
- ❑ D sodium bicarbonate must be given to prevent acidosis
- ❑ E calcium chloride is recommended for asystole

1.42 The following diseases and antibodies are associated:

		Antibody	*Disease*
❑	A	antimitochondrial	CREST
❑	B	rheumatoid factor	rheumatoid arthritis
❑	C	anti double-stranded DNA	SLE
❑	D	anticardiolipin	SLE
❑	E	anti centromere	primary biliary cirrhosis

1.43 The following apply to the management of chronic obstructive pulmonary disease (COPD):

- ❑ A in the treatment of an exacerbation, 24% oxygen should be used initially
- ❑ B long-term oxygen has been shown to improve life expectancy
- ❑ C influenza vaccine is contraindicated
- ❑ D in an infective exacerbation the most likely organism is *Staphylococcus aureus*
- ❑ E regular blood transfusions may help to increase oxygen carrying capacity

1.44 Spontaneous rib fracture may be caused by

- ❑ A coughing
- ❑ B metastases
- ❑ C primary lung tumour
- ❑ D pneumothorax
- ❑ E osteoporosis

1.45 Rapid respiration may be caused by

- ❑ A hyperosmolar ketoacidosis
- ❑ B salicylate overdose
- ❑ C hypoglycaemia
- ❑ D lesions of the pons
- ❑ E anxiety

1.46 The following are causes of a pleural effusion:

- ❑ A pancreatitis
- ❑ B ovarian carcinoma
- ❑ C retroperitoneal fibrosis
- ❑ D mesothelioma
- ❑ E pulmonary infarction

1.47 The following are associated with dilatation of the pupil:

- ❑ A complete third nerve palsy
- ❑ B Horner's syndrome
- ❑ C entering the garden on a bright day
- ❑ D old age
- ❑ E convergence

1.48 Spontaneous pneumothorax

- ❑ A usually occurs in men
- ❑ B is best treated with positive pressure ventilation
- ❑ C may be managed by observation alone
- ❑ D if left alone, a 100% pneumothorax would take 2–3 weeks to fully re-expand
- ❑ E is often caused by rib fractures

1.49 Recognised features of sarcoidosis include

- ❑ A lymphocytosis
- ❑ B lupus pernio
- ❑ C facial nerve palsy
- ❑ D splenomegaly
- ❑ E bilateral hilar lymphadenopathy

1.50 The following can be attributed to a urinary tract infection in an elderly person:

- ❑ A falls
- ❑ B disorientation
- ❑ C urinary incontinence
- ❑ D anaemia
- ❑ E wandering at night

1.51 Portosystemic encephalopathy may be precipitated by

- ❑ A gastrointestinal haemorrhage
- ❑ B lactulose
- ❑ C benzodiazepines
- ❑ D diuretics
- ❑ E constipation

1.52 The following apply to the arterial blood pressure:

- ❑ A on standing the systolic and diastolic pressures rise
- ❑ B it increases on exercise
- ❑ C there is a diurnal variation
- ❑ D there may be a difference between the right and left brachial pressures
- ❑ E it is falsely high when a small cuff is used

1.53 Causes of a collapsing pulse include

- ❑ A aortic regurgitation
- ❑ B thyrotoxicosis
- ❑ C mitral stenosis
- ❑ D bradycardia
- ❑ E fever

1.54 The following statements on mortality rates are true:

❑ A the maternal mortality rate is the number of deaths of mothers attributable to pregnancy and delivery divided by the number of births
❑ B the perinatal mortality rate is the number of deaths in the first week of life (excluding stillbirths) divided by the total number of births
❑ C the neonatal mortality rate is the number of deaths in the first four weeks of life divided by the number of deaths in the first year
❑ D the stillbirth rate is the number of babies born dead after 28 weeks divided by the number of live births
❑ E the infant mortality rate is the number of deaths in the first year divided by the number of live births

1.55 The following apply to infectious diseases:

❑ A since 1992 there has been a reduction in the incidence of *Haemophilus influenzae* type B infections in children
❑ B there have been no confirmed cases of measles since 1994
❑ C smallpox was declared to have been eradicated from the world in the 1960s
❑ D *H. influenzae* type B viruses are subject to antigenic shift
❑ E approximately 90% of adults are immune to chickenpox

1.56 Immunisation is the main factor responsible for the reduction in rates of

❑ A pulmonary tuberculosis
❑ B diphtheria
❑ C whooping cough
❑ D cholera
❑ E measles

1.57 The following are side effects of inhaled steroids:

❑ A cataracts
❑ B oral candidiasis
❑ C hoarse voice
❑ D Cushing's disease
❑ E adrenal suppression

1.58 Polyuria may result from

- ❑ A hypokalaemia
- ❑ B hypercalcaemia
- ❑ C an epileptic attack
- ❑ D diabetes insipidus
- ❑ E hypoglycaemia

1.59 The following statements about systolic murmurs are true:

- ❑ A mitral valve prolapse produces a pansystolic murmur
- ❑ B the murmur of a ventricular septal defect is pansystolic
- ❑ C hypertrophic obstructive cardiomyopathy produces a murmur loudest on squatting
- ❑ D an atrial septal defect produces an ejection systolic murmur
- ❑ E aortic stenosis produces an early systolic murmur

1.60 Leucocytes in the urine occur with

- ❑ A aspirin nephropathy
- ❑ B nephroblastoma
- ❑ C renal tuberculosis
- ❑ D retroperitoneal fibrosis
- ❑ E polycystic renal disease

END

Go over your answers until your time is up.
Correct answers and teaching notes are overleaf.

MULTIPLE CHOICE QUESTION PAPER 1 – ANSWERS

The correct answer options for each question are given below.

1.1	All false
1.2	A D
1.3	A C
1.4	A B C D
1.5	D
1.6	A D
1.7	A C D
1.8	A
1.9	A C D E
1.10	All false
1.11	C D
1.12	C D
1.13	A B C D
1.14	A B D E
1.15	B C
1.16	A B C
1.17	A B C D
1.18	D E
1.19	A B C D
1.20	A C D E
1.21	A B D E
1.22	A B C E
1.23	C E
1.24	A B
1.25	B C D E
1.26	C E
1.27	A B
1.28	A B C D
1.29	A C D E
1.30	A B C D E
1.31	C D E
1.32	A B
1.33	C
1.34	A B E
1.35	D
1.36	A
1.37	A B E
1.38	A B C
1.39	A B C D E
1.40	A E
1.41	B C
1.42	B C D
1.43	A B
1.44	A B C E
1.45	A B D E
1.46	A B D E
1.47	A
1.48	A C
1.49	A B C D E
1.50	A B C
1.51	A C D E
1.52	B C D E
1.53	A B E
1.54	A E
1.55	A B E
1.56	B C E
1.57	B C E
1.58	A B D
1.59	B C D
1.60	A B C

MCQ PAPER 1 – ANSWERS AND TEACHING NOTES

1.1 Deep vein thrombosis — Answers: All false

Deep vein thromboses are common, particularly in immobile patients such as fractured neck of femur. 20% of deep vein thromboses extend proximally and approximately 2% embolise. A duplex ultrasound is the first line investigation. A venogram should not be performed routinely as it is more invasive and involves a radiation dose to the patient.

The use of low molecular weight heparin injections which can be given by a district nurse have made outpatient treatment preferable. Admission is however advised for the following conditions:

- increased risk of bleeding
- bilateral deep vein thromboses
- extension to the inferior vena cava
- pulmonary embolus
- dementia
- intravenous drug abuse

An above knee deep vein thrombosis should be treated with 6 months of anticoagulation. Three months of treatment is advised if the thrombus is at the trifurcation i.e. where the three main veins of the leg join to form the popliteal vein.

A below knee deep vein thrombosis may cause clinical problems such as skin changes from venous obstruction. A pulmonary embolus is extremely unlikely and the risks of anticoagulation outweigh the risk of pulmonary embolus.

1.2 Pulmonary embolism — Answers: A D

A pulmonary embolism is unlikely if the arterial oxygen is above 10.7 kPa or if the respiratory rate is <20 respirations per minute. The chest X-ray is often normal in a patient with a pulmonary embolus. D-Dimer measurements are useful. If the D-Dimer levels are below 0.3 ml/l an acute pulmonary embolus is unlikely. Note that a raised D-Dimer is not diagnostic because it is elevated in malignant disease, infection, recent surgery and if the total bilirubin is above 34 ml/l.

Pulmonary embolism occurs in young adults. Those with increased risk are women on the contraceptive pill; patients with a family history of thrombosis, patients who have undergone recent surgery, trauma, immobilisation or who have a malignancy.

1.3 Asthma **Answers: A C**

The features of severe asthma include:

- a peak flow <50 % of the patient's best measurement or predicted
- tachycardia >110 beats per minutes irrespective of whether a beta-agonist has been given
- tachypnoea >25 respirations/minute
- unable to complete a whole sentence

A potentially fatal asthmatic attack is indicated by:

- a peak flow of <33%
- cyanosis/hypoxia
- a silent chest on osculation – it is important to remember that if no wheeze can be heard this is a bad sign as it implies that air entry into the chest is so poor that a wheeze cannot be generated. Do not interpret the absence of a wheeze to mean that there is no broncho-constriction
- PCO_2 > 6 KPa suggests fatigue and imminent respiratory failure – the PCO_2 should be low because of hyperventilation
- a previous ITU admission indicates that the patient is prone to life threatening attacks

Acute asthma still carries a high mortality. In the United Kingdom approximately 2,000 people die from this each year. Always remember to have a low threshold for contacting an anaesthetist to ventilate the patient.

1.4 Blood pressure **Answers: A B C D**

Patients must be admitted and treated in hospital if the raised blood pressure is causing end organ damage, e.g. retinal damage, renal damage, encephalopathy, seizures or coma. Myocardial infarction, dissecting aneurysm and pulmonary oedema may also be caused by a severe rise in blood pressure and are also indications of urgent treatment. Note the blood pressure should be brought down slowly aiming for a diastolic blood pressure of around 110–115 mmHg after 24 hours. A sudden drop in blood pressure may precipitate myocardial infarction, stroke and acute renal failure. Intravenous therapy should therefore be avoided and if it is necessary should be given in an ITU setting.

1.5 ECG changes **Answer: D**

Diagnostic features of acute myocardial infarction are:

- ST elevation greater than or equal to 1 mm in two adjacent limbs lead
- ST elevation of greater than or equal to 2 mm in two adjacent precordial leads
- Left bundle branch block that is new in the context of a convincing history

Note that if there is a convincing history then any ST elevation may be significant but before thrombolysis the case should be discussed with a senior doctor.

1.6 Contraindications to thrombolysis **Answers: A D**

There are major and relative contraindications to thrombolysis. If any of these are present the case should be discussed urgently with a senior doctor, such as the on-call cardiology registrar.

The major contraindications to thrombolysis are active bleeding or known bleeding disorders and the following specific conditions:

- CNS: previous subarachnoid or intra-cerebral bleed, haemorrhagic stroke, neoplasm aneurysm or AV malformation. A recent stroke within one year; head injury or CNS surgery within six months.
- Cardiac: suspected aortic dissection. Traumatic cardio-pulmonary resuscitation within one month.
- GI: acute pancreatitis, oesophageal varices, any recent major surgery or bleeding within two months.
- Obstetric: pregnancy; obstetric delivery within 10 days/heavy vaginal bleeding (but not a normal menstruation).
- Orthopaedic: bone fracture within one month.

  The relative contraindications are
- CNS: history of stroke with residual deficit, proliferative diabetic retinopathy/laser treatment.
- Cardiac: a blood pressure of >200/110 mmHg; this should be treated first. Puncture of a non-compressible artery within two weeks.
- GI: active peptic ulcer disease. Organ biopsy in the last two weeks. Tooth extraction within the last month.
- Respiratory: cavitating pulmonary disease
- Oral anticoagulant therapy is a relative contraindication, as is any minor surgery within the last month.

1.7 Abdominal X-ray **Answers: A C D**

Under normal circumstances there is a large amount of gas in the large bowel, a great deal less in the small bowel. The small bowel tends to lie centrally. The ascending and descending colon are normally the most laterally seen loops of bowel. The transverse colon is usually identified crossing the upper abdomen.

In the small bowel the valvulae conniventes are seen as parallel bands, extending fully across the lumen. They are particularly noticeable when the small bowel is distended. Small bowel is abnormally distended if the loops are >3 cm in diameter. The large bowel has haustral folds that extend only one-third across the lumen. The large bowel is dilated if > 5.5 cm in diameter.

1.8 Unstable angina **Answer: A**

Unstable angina is a term that many cardiologists no longer use. The term was used to describe the clinical syndrome of rapidly worsening, prolonged or increasingly frequent episodes of chest pain, or pain occurring at rest or chest pain of recent onset. Many cardiologists use the term 'acute coronary syndrome' which encompasses the spectrum of conditions with mild ischaemia at one end of the spectrum and myocardial infarction at the other end. The risk of myocardial infarction or death within six weeks of developing the above conditions may be as high as 10% and the condition must therefore be taken seriously. The patient must be admitted to hospital and ideally to the Coronary Care Unit. Observation and continuous ECG monitoring should be performed. Intravenous access and blood sample for cardiac troponin levels should also be performed. The treatment involves aspirin, subcutaneous low molecular weight heparin, intravenous nitrates, beta-blockade. In patients with unstable angina and high risk coronary anatomy – there is a case for giving a glycoprotein IIB IIIA receptor antagonist such as abciximab and the case should be discussed with the on-call cardiologist. The cardiologist should also be contacted to discuss patients who fail to improve on the above treatment so that urgent coronary angiography can be considered.
Cardiac troponin is highly specific for cardiac damage.

1.9 Gastro-intestinal bleed **Answers: A C D E**

It is useful to divide patients into high and low risk groups to determine management. A patient is high risk if they are hypotensive, there has been a haematemesis or melaena has been passed, tachycardia >100, postural hypotension and co-morbidity.

The patient is deemed to be low risk if they are <60 years of age, they have had a coffee-ground vomitus and the cardiovascular parameters are stable. Low risk patients should be admitted and given fluids. They should be observed for signs of further bleeding and an endoscopy should be booked for the next routine list.

Patients at high risk who are unstable e.g. with hypotension require immediate resuscitation and urgent endoscopy in the presence of a surgeon. Patients who are at high risk but who are stable require resuscitation and should have an endoscopy with 12 hours.

1.10 Acute asthma **Answers: All false**

The treatment of acute asthma is as follows:

- Oxygen: a high concentration of 6l/min is required as most patients will have a low PCO_2. The issue of low concentration oxygen is only relevant in CO_2 retaining patients with COPD (chronic obstructive pulmonary disease).
- Broncho-dilators: oxygen driven nebulised broncho-dilators such as salbutamol should be started as soon as possible. If there is no improvement these should be repeated at 15 minute intervals. Nebulised ipratropium bromide helps in about 30% of patients and can be given every six hours.
- An IV broncho-dilator should only be given if the patient has failed to respond to repeated nebulised treatment.
- Corticosteroids: these should be given as soon as possible as they take six hours to produce improvement. Intravenous hydrocortisone 200 ml or prednisolone 60 ml orally may be given.
- Magnesium: for patients with severe asthma who respond poorly to nebulised broncho-dilators, intravenous magnesium may be given as an infusion. Note the question says oral magnesium and is therefore false.
- Aminophylline: this is rarely given now because of limited efficacy and numerous side effects.
- Hydration: patients are often dehydrated as they have not been drinking enough because of being unwell and also via extra loss through hyperventilation. Patients should be rehydrated with intravenous fluids.

  Chest X-ray: this should be done to exclude a pneumo-thorax and to look for supra added infection.

1.11 Jugular venous pressure **Answers: C D**

The A wave is due to atrial contraction. The V wave is due to venous return to the right atrium during ventricular systole. Large A waves are due to increased atrial contraction, for example, in tricuspid stenosis, pulmonary stenosis and pulmonary hypertension. Tricuspid stenosis causes large A waves but not cannon waves. Cannon waves occur when the right ventricle and atrium contract simultaneously, as in complete heart block or ventricular tachycardia.

The jugular venous pressure (JVP) is raised in congestive cardiac failure but not in pure left ventricular failure.

During inspiration intrathoracic pressure falls, causing blood to be sucked into the right side of the heart. This is responsible for the normal fall in JVP on inspiration. If the right side of the heart is physically prevented from relaxing to accommodate the increase in venous return the venous pressure rises. This occurs in constrictive pericarditis and cardiac tamponade and this paradoxical rise in the JVP is known as Kussmaul's sign.

In tricuspid regurgitation large V waves and a pulsatile liver are features, but the mitral valve is on the LEFT side and therefore has no effect on the JVP.

1.12 Cerebellar lesions **Answers: C D**

The features of a cerebellar syndrome may be remembered by the mnemonic *DANISH:*

- **D**ysdiadochokinesis
- **A**taxia (patients have a broad-based gait with a tendency to fall to the side of the lesion. They are unable to walk heel to toe)
- **N**ystagmus
- **I**ntention tremor
- **S**lurred speech
- **H**ypotonia

The plantar responses are typically flexor and the neurological signs are ipsilateral as the majority of pathways from the cerebellum do not cross over.

1.13 Gastrointestinal malignancy Answers: A B C D

This is an extremely common question that has been seen in both general medicine and paediatric sections and also in general surgery papers. The stems that have been reported most frequently are C, E and A (in that order).

Familial adenomatous polyposis coli is caused by an autosomal dominant gene on chromosome 5. Multiple polyps occur in the colon during adolescence, and carcinoma typically develops in the third decade. This condition accounts for 1% of all cases of colon cancer.

Recent evidence suggests that *H. pylori* infection increases the risk of gastric lymphoma. Regression of the lymphoma is said to occur on eradication of the infection. Gastric adenocarcinoma is also associated with *H. pylori.*

Coeliac disease causes increased risk of small-bowel lymphoma. When a patient's symptoms persist, despite adhering to a strict gluten-free diet, the development of lymphoma should be strongly suspected. There is also an increased risk of oesophageal carcinoma with coeliac disease.

Peutz-Jeghers syndrome is characterised by buccal pigmentation and small bowel polyps which are non-malignant. Inheritance is autosomal dominant. A few textbooks argue that the polyps have some malignant potential, and there is some evidence of an increase in upper gastrointestinal tract malignancy.

Uncomplicated reflux does not cause malignancy. A condition such as Barrett's oesophagus, which is associated with chronic reflux, does however increase the risk of oesophageal carcinoma.

The risk of oesophageal cancer is also increased in achalasia and in Plummer-Vinson (Patterson-Brown-Kelly) syndrome, the condition of iron deficiency in association with an oesophageal web.

1.14 Benign intracranial hypertension Answers: A B D E

This condition is more common in obese young women especially if taking drugs such as the oral contraceptive pill, tetracyclines and retinoids. Benign intracranial hypertension (BIH) causes marked papilloedema and can cause blindness. Headaches are a frequent symptom and are caused by the raised intracranial pressure. They improve dramatically post-lumbar puncture that forms the basis of treatment. The carbonic anhydrase inhibitor acetazolamide is also used. When these methods fail, shunts can be inserted surgically.

1.15 Gynaecomastia **Answers: B C**

This is a very common question.

Gynaecomastia refers to enlargement of the male breast due to an increase in breast tissue. Oestrogen is the main hormone responsible for this and hence oestrogen-secreting tumours, such as testicular tumours and certain types of bronchial carcinoma, may cause gynaecomastia. Oestrogen is normally metabolised by the liver and so its levels are increased in liver failure. In chronic renal failure altered hormone binding produces a functional excess of oestrogen.

Human chorionic gonadotrophin (HCG) secretion also causes gynaecomastia. Testicular tumours can therefore produce gynaecomastia by production of oestrogen or HCG.

It is a common misconception that prolactin increases breast tissue growth. This is not the case. Hyper-prolactinaemia, however, may cause galactorrhoea (i.e. milk production and secretion) but do not confuse this with gynaecomastia.

Drug causes of gynaecomastia include cimetidine, spironolactone and digoxin.

1.16 Peptic ulceration **Answers: A B C**

Duodenal ulcers do not become malignant. This is in contrast to gastric ulcers that may be malignant and must therefore be biopsied at endoscopy. Gastric ulceration is thought to be due to lowered mucosal resistance whereas duodenal ulcers are usually associated with increased acid production.

Helicobacter pylori is associated with:

- duodenal ulceration (95%)
- gastric ulceration (75%)
- chronic antral gastritis (90%)

1.17 Erythema nodosum **Answers: A B C D**

Erythema nodosum is a painful rash usually occurring on the lower leg but it may also occur on the forearm. It is produced by conditions that cause a subcutaneous vasculitis. Causes include any streptococcal infection, acute sarcoidosis, tuberculosis, inflammatory bowel disease, pregnancy, leprosy, Behçet's disease and syphilis.

Drugs that may cause erythema nodosum include penicillin, oral contraceptives, codeine, salicylates and barbiturates.

1.18 Urine testing **Answers: D E**

Normal urine contains <20 mg/l of albumin. A dipstick detects > 150 mg/l. The level between the two is known as microalbuminuria and it is an early indicator of diabetic nephropathy.

Urine dipsticks can detect blood and the presence of white cells, but only microscopy detects casts (read the question carefully!).

Dipsticks are relatively insensitive to globulin and Bence-Jones proteins. White cells indicate inflammation/infection.

Nitrite is due to bacterial metabolism. Its absence does not exclude infection, but its presence on dipstick testing indicates infection with a specificity of 95%.

1.19 Goitre **Answers: A B C D**

Pregnancy and puberty are both physiological causes of a goitre.
In Graves' disease the gland is diffusely enlarged, firm and often associated with a bruit.

Excess doses of carbimazole induce goitre.

Exogenous iodine inhibits TSH release and thus the stimulus for thyroid gland hypertrophy. Hence, in areas of iodine deficiency, people may develop a goitre.

Items D and E are often incorrectly answered.

1.20 Syncope **Answers: A C D E**

This is a very common question and may be found in both the adult and paediatric sections. Pertussis infection causes episodes of persistent coughing and anoxia that can result in syncope.

Menière's disease causes vertigo, tinnitus and deafness but not true syncope. HOCM may result in such marked ventricular hypertrophy as to cause obstruction to cardiac outflow.

Always remember *any* arrhythmia can cause syncope.

1.21 Glycosuria **Answers: A B D E**

One per cent of the population has a low renal threshold for glucose. Glucocorticoids and growth hormone increase blood glucose levels and may produce hyperglycaemia. Conversely, Addison's disease may cause hypoglycaemia.

In Fanconi syndrome amino acids are also excreted in the urine due to a generalised proximal tubular defect.

Growth hormone has a diabetogenic effect.

Do not be misled by the word 'may' and mark item C as true.

1.22 Diarrhoea **Answers: A B C E**

The definition of diarrhoea is the passage of loose stools in excess of 300 g in 24 hours. It is useful to divide the causes into whether the stool is:

- Watery
  Dietary indiscretions
  Infections, e.g. cholera, rotavirus
  Metabolic, e.g. hyperthyroidism, hypocalcaemia, Addison's disease, carcinoid syndrome
  Diabetic autonomic neuropathy produces diarrhoea especially nocturnal.
  Note: Addison's disease may also cause constipation, as may hypothyroidism, and hypercalcemia (hence D is false).

- Bloody
  Inflammatory bowel disease
  Bowel malignancy
  Infection, e.g. Salmonella, Shigella, *Clostridium difficile*

- Steatorrhoea
  Small bowel malabsorption
  Pancreatic disease

1.23 Hypercalcaemia **Answers: C E**

The most common causes of hypercalcaemia are hyperparathyroidism and malignancy.

In sarcoidosis non-caseating granulomas form. These contain activated macrophages which produce a PTH related peptide resulting in hypercalcemia.

The raised calcium levels produced by sarcoidosis, multiple myeloma and vitamin D toxicity are typically steroid suppressible.

Other causes include benign familial hypercalcaemia, thyrotoxicosis, hypothyroidism in infants, phaeochromocytoma, and drugs such as lithium and thiazide diuretics.

Pseudohypoparathyroidism is caused by end organ resistance to PTH. It is associated with short stature, short metacarpals and intellectual impairment. It is called 'pseudo' because there is a biochemical picture of hypoparathyroidism with low calcium and high phosphate, although in fact the PTH is not low but is appropriately high.

Pseudopseudohypoparathyroidism is so called because it produces phenotypic features of pseudohypoparathyroidism but without calcium abnormality.

Acute pancreatitis causes hypocalcaemia because of extensive fat necrosis.

Paget's disease causes increased bone turnover. Calcium and phosphate are normal but alkaline phosphatase is elevated. However, after a period of immobilisation calcium levels may rise.

1.24 Normal chest X-ray Answers: A B

The right hemidiaphragm is higher than the left because it is 'pushed' up by the liver.

The left hilum is higher than the right.

The right main bronchus is lower, shorter, wider and more vertical than the left and hence inhaled foreign bodies (e.g. peanuts) may lodge in it.

The lower end of the trachea is slightly to the right of the midline. The right lung consists of three lobes. The upper and middle lobes are anterior and are separated from each other by the horizontal fissure. The oblique fissure demarcates the lower lobe that lies posteriorly. In the left lung, only the upper (anterior) and lower (posterior) lobes are present, separated from each other by the oblique fissure.

Magnification of the heart occurs in an AP and a portable film. This is because the film is behind the patient's back and the X-rays shone from the front produce a wider angle to reach it.

1.25 Papilloedema Answers: B C D E

Causes of papilloedema can be divided as follows:

- Raised intracranial pressure
  Space-occupying lesion (tumour, cerebral abscess); benign intracranial hypertension (OCP, retinoids, tetracyclines); hypertensive encephalopathy; hypercapnia; venous sinus thrombosis.
- Accelerated phase hypertension (malignant hypertension)
- Retinal vein obstruction
  Tumour; cortical venous sinus thrombosis; central retinal vein thrombosis.
- Miscellaneous (rare)
  Metabolic: hypercapnia, vitamin A poisoning, lead poisoning.
  Endocrine: hypoparathyroidism, exophthalmos.
  Haematological: sudden/severe anaemia.
  Infection: subacute bacterial endocarditis.

1.26 Cystic fibrosis **Answers: C E**

Cystic fibrosis is an important autosomal recessive condition which occurs in 1 in 2000 live births. The most common mutation responsible is found on the delta F508 region of chromosome 7. Screening for the carrier status is possible and prenatal diagnosis by amniocentesis is possible.

Presentation may be with bowel obstruction due to meconium ileus in babies or meconium ileus equivalent at an older age. Frequent respiratory tract infections with the development of bronchiectasis or simply a failure to thrive should lead to a suspicion of the diagnosis.

The defect is due to an abnormality of chloride ion transport and the resulting excess of sodium loss in the sweat forms the basis of the sweat test for cystic fibrosis. Many body secretions become abnormally viscous; for example, in the lung predisposing to infection, and also in the pancreas leading to malabsorption and an increased risk of diabetes mellitus. The thickened bowel secretions and steatorrhoea predispose to bowel obstruction (meconium ileus equivalent). This can be made worse by surgery and should be treated conservatively. Liver cirrhosis with portal hypertension may develop.

In the male the vas deferens is absent and so although sperm production is virtually normal its transport is not, resulting in infertility.

The mainstay of treatment is regular physiotherapy with postural drainage, early use of antibiotics during infective exacerbations, and pancreatic enzyme replacement. Nebulised DNase is of use in thinning lung secretions. Gene therapy using liposomes and viruses as vectors to carry the normal gene is at an experimental stage. Most patients survive well into adulthood.

1.27 Pulmonary embolism **Answers: A B**

Other options which might occur with this question include:

• Pulsus paradoxus	True; see overleaf
• Deep venous thrombosis	False; a DVT may cause a pulmonary embolism, but not vice versa
• Heparin treatment should only be started when a positive VQ scan result is obtained	False; see overleaf

Pulmonary embolism may be mild or severe, single or multiple.

Although it may be asymptomatic, it usually produces pleuritic chest pain, tachypnoea and tachycardia. The JVP may be elevated and a pulsus paradoxus may be present.

In any patient with a cough, haemoptysis or hypotension a pulmonary embolus must be considered.

Hypoxia occurs and the oxygen saturation falls. Hyperventilation produces a fall in PCO_2.

The most common ECG finding is a sinus tachycardia. Signs of right heart strain including RBBB may also occur. The classic S1 Q3 T3 (an S wave in V1, Q wave in lead III and T wave inversion in lead III) is uncommon.
The chest X-ray is often normal but a small pleural effusion may occur. Band shadows from atelectasis occur in both infection and infarction. Wedge-shaped peripheral consolidation may also occur.

If a pulmonary embolism is suspected the patient should be given heparin (providing there are no contraindications) before obtaining a VQ scan. Treatment also involves giving oxygen and appropriate analgesia.

A ventilation perfusion scan compares the distribution of blood flow with the parts of the lung being ventilated. When a blood clot lodges in a major blood vessel, blood is diverted from it to other vessels creating a perfusion defect. Ventilation is usually unaffected leading to a mismatched defect in ventilation and perfusion. Spiral CT with intravenous contrast using a pulmonary angiogram protocol is very sensitive in the diagnosis of a pulmonary embolus.

1.28 Dysphagia **Answers: A B C D**

Dysphagia literally means difficulty with swallowing. It does not necessarily imply there is pain or vomiting, although these may coexist.
There may be a physical obstruction in the lumen of the oesophagus, for example, oesophageal carcinoma or a benign peptic stricture.
Disorders of the muscle wall and/or its nerve supply may also produce dysphagia, for example:

- pseudo-bulbar palsy: bilateral stroke
- bulbar palsy: motor neurone disease, Guillain-Barré syndrome, polio, myasthenia gravis

- autonomic plexus disorders: achalasia, Chagas'disease, Guillain-Barré syndrome.

Anxiety may cause globus hystericus.
Pyloric stenosis produces projectile vomiting but not dysphagia.

1.29 Acromegaly **Answers: A C D E**

Acromegaly is produced by an excess of growth hormone. Before puberty, excess growth hormone produces the syndrome of gigantism. After the epiphyses have fused an increase in height does not occur but instead there is an overgrowth of organs and soft tissue. The face is enlarged with prominent supraorbital ridges, enlarged jaw (prognathism), widely spaced teeth and poor occlusion of the teeth when the mouth closes. The tongue is large. The hands are enlarged and spade-like; they have a doughy feel to them and the skin is greasy.

The pituitary macroadenoma that is usually responsible may cause compression of the optic chiasm producing a visual field defect. This is usually a bilateral hemianopia, but an upper outer quadrantanopia may be an early sign. Optic atrophy may occur but blindness is not a common feature of acromegaly.

Other organs increase in size and hepatosplenomegaly may occur. An increase in heart size may produce a cardiomyopathy. Soft tissue overgrowth may cause compression of nerves, for example the median nerve, producing carpal tunnel syndrome. Arthropathy is also a feature.
Hypertension is common and as growth hormone causes an increase in blood glucose, diabetes mellitus may also result.

It is said that one-third of patients present because of symptoms, one-third because they notice a change in their appearance and one-third are noticed by their doctors to have a change in appearance.

The important features may be remembered as follows:
A Arthropathy
B Blood pressure (increase)
C Carpal tunnel syndrome
D Diabetes mellitus
E Enlargement (of organs, face, hands and feet)
F Field defect (bitemporal hemianopia)

1.30 Osteoporosis **Answers: A B C D E**

Osteoporosis is a condition where a reduction in bone density occurs, predisposing to fractures. The bone constituents are normal but reduced. Serum calcium, phosphate and alkaline phosphatase are normal.

Bone formation/remodelling is dependent on normal movement, metabolic factors and hormones. Metabolic disorders, such as thyrotoxicosis, Cushing's syndrome and steroid therapy, cause this reduction in bone mass.

Oestrogen promotes bone growth, and deficiency states, such as the menopause, are important risk factors. HRT not only prevents further bone loss but can promote bone regeneration. In a recent study, bone mineral content increased by 3.7% in patients on HRT while a decrease of 5.7% occurred in those on placebo. (Bone mass in post-menopausal women after withdrawal of oestrogen/ gestagen replacement therapy. Christiansen C. et al. *Lancet*, 1981; 1 (8218): 459-461.)

In prolonged immobilisation the local stress/strain on bone is absent; remodelling does not occur, increasing the risk of osteoporosis. A low body weight, for example in athletes and those with anorexia nervosa, also predispose to it and genetic and racial factors are important. (Asians and Orientals have a higher incidence.) The incidence also rises with age and is more common in women; by the age of 70 a woman will have lost 50% of her bone mass and one in two women will have sustained an osteoporotic fracture.

1.31 Ocular complications of diabetes mellitus **Answers: C D E**

The most common form of diabetic eye disease is diabetic retinopathy which is classified as follows:

- Background retinopathy
  (1) Dot haemorrhages which are actually capillary microaneurysms
  (2) Blot haemorrhages which are caused by leakage of blood into the deeper layers of the retina
  (3) Hard exudates which are bright yellow/white clearly defined lesions caused by exudates of lipid and protein. These changes take at least 10 years to develop.
- Maculopathy
  More commonly seen in NIDDM. Hard exudates appear in a circular pattern around the macula; a serious complication, as visual acuity may decline rapidly.

- Pre-proliferative retinopathy
  The following are classified as pre-proliferative changes as they are thought to induce proliferative changes:
  (1) Cotton wool spots (soft exudates) which are patches of retinal oedema caused by ischaemia
  (2) Venous beading/looping
  (3) More than three blot haemorrhages
- Proliferative retinopathy
  Hypoxia is thought to be the signal for new vessel formation. These new vessels are fragile and haemorrhage easily. This encourages fibrous proliferation producing traction bands and eventually retinal detachment. Fifty per cent of these patients will be blind in five years.
- Cataracts
  More common with advancing age; juvenile/snowflake cataracts are diffuse rapidly progressive cataracts associated with poorly controlled diabetes mellitus.
- Glaucoma
  Diabetics have an increased risk of acute glaucoma due to rubeosis iridis (new vessel formation at the iris blocks fluid drainage at the canal of Schlemm leading to a sudden increase in intraocular pressure).
  There is also an increased incidence of chronic glaucoma.
- Cranial nerve palsy – especially III.

1.32 Primary hyperaldosteronism — Answers: A B

This question requires a knowledge of the biochemistry of primary hyperaldosteronism:

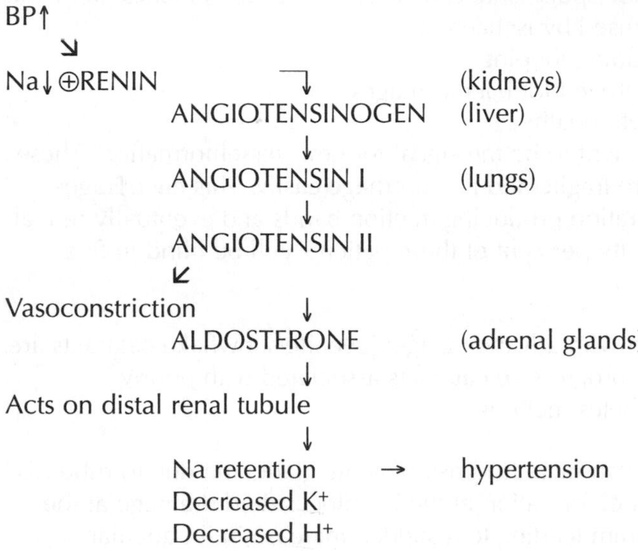

Aldosterone increases sodium reabsorption in exchange for potassium and hydrogen in the distal renal tubule, resulting in a hypernatraemic hypokalaemic metabolic alkalosis.

Renin levels are low because of negative feedback by increased aldosterone.

Salt and water retention produce hypertension.

1.33 Insulin-dependent diabetes mellitus — Answer: C

Diabetic nephropathy affects 25–30% of diabetic patients. Patients with diabetic renal disease will almost certainly also have some degree of retinopathy, but the converse is not true. Diabetic retinopathy is much more common than nephropathy.

Maculopathy is more common in Type II diabetes mellitus.

Pre-proliferative and proliferative retinopathy is most commonly found in Type I diabetes mellitus.

The aetiology of diabetes mellitus is complex. An increased susceptibility may be inherited, with the greatest risk if the father is diabetic.

Ninety-five per cent of IDDM patients carry HLA DR3, HLA DR4 or both. Interestingly, people with HLA DR2 have a reduced risk.
Viruses – *Coxsackie type B4.*

The main problem in Type I diabetes is a lack of insulin, whereas in Type II insulin is present but there is a peripheral resistance to it. During illness the stress hormones (e.g. cortisol) increase causing hyperglycaemia and increasing insulin requirements.

1.34 Nephrotic syndrome **Answers: A B E**

The definition of nephrotic syndrome comprises:

- proteinuria of 3–5 g over 24 hours
- hypoalbuminuria
- peripheral oedema

It is also associated with a hypercoagulable state and hypercholesterolaemia but this is not strictly in the formal definition. There are many causes:

- Congenital
- Acquired:
  Glomerulonephritis (most commonly minimal change, focal sclerosing, membranous)
  Diabetes
  Systemic vasculitis, especially SLE drugs (e.g. gold, penicillamine)
  Infection (e.g. malaria)
  Myeloma
  Allergies

Interstitial nephritis, as the name implies, causes a nephritis rather than a nephrotic syndrome. Nephritis produces much less proteinuria and causes haematuria that is usually microscopic.

This question appears frequently. Other options to bear in mind are renal papillary necrosis, chronic tubulointerstitial nephritis, renal TB and polycystic renal disease. All may cause proteinuria but not enough to cause the syndrome that – remember – has a strict definition.

1.35 Paget's disease **Answer: D**

In Paget's disease there is increased resorption of bone due to increased osteoclastic activity and secondary abnormal bone formation. Patients may be remarkably asymptomatic despite extensive skeletal involvement. Clinical features include bone pain and local tenderness, bone deformity and fractures. The skull is enlarged and the bony overgrowth may produce cranial nerve damage: for example, optic atrophy, and deafness. The latter may also be caused by overgrowth of the ossicles. High output cardiac failure may occur and although everyone remembers the complication of osteosarcoma, note that it only occurs in 1–2% of patients. Remember *PANICS:*

Pain
Arthritis
Nerve compression
Increased bone size
Cardiac failure
Sarcoma

Diagnosis is made by history, examination and investigations.

Bone turnover is increased resulting in a raised alkaline phosphatase. Although bone is resorbed it is also reformed and so serum calcium and phosphate are normal (recent immobilization may cause hypercalcaemia). X-rays show disorganised bone, with bony expansion and a coarsened trabecular pattern. Treatment includes pain relief, calcitonin, sodium etidronate and treatment of complications.

1.36 Diabetes mellitus **Answer: A**

This is a very difficult question. Remember the WHO criteria for the diagnosis of diabetes mellitus:

	Plasma	Whole blood
Fasting glucose	>7.8	>6.7
Random glucose	>11.1	>10.0

Whole blood values are 1.1 less than plasma because the red blood cells use up glucose. Ideally, two abnormal values should be obtained. When a value between 7.8–11.1 or 6.7–10 occurs then a 75 g glucose tolerance test should be performed. A fasting plasma glucose ≥7.8 or a two-hour value ≥11.1 is diagnostic. Values in between imply impaired glucose tolerance, and a proportion of these people will go on to develop diabetes mellitus.

Islet cell antibodies are of interest because they provide evidence for an autoimmune aetiology, but they are not currently used in routine diagnosis.

Glycosuria reflects the degree of diabetic control, but 1% of the population and pregnant women have a low renal threshold for glucose reabsorption and so glycosuria is suggestive of diabetes mellitus but is not diagnostic. Retinal new vessel formation occurs in response to hypoxia of any aetiology, for example sickle cell disease.

1.37 Ptosis **Answers: A B E**

A ptosis is a drooping eyelid and may be complete (the eye is closed) or partial. It may be unilateral or bilateral.
Damage at any of the following sites will result in a ptosis:

- III nerve damage: posterior communicating artery aneurysm mid-brain lesion
- Sympathetic nerve damage: Horner's syndrome
- Muscle/neuromuscular nerve junction: dystrophia myotonica (usually bilateral) myasthenia gravis (ptosis is fatiguable and often bilateral).

Parasympathetic damage itself does not cause a ptosis. See Paper 1, Question 47 on pupil dilation for details.

Note that a VII nerve palsy results in an inability to close the eye. *It never causes a ptosis.*

1.38 Bell's palsy **Answers: A B C**

A Bell's palsy is a common, acute, isolated facial nerve palsy. Damage to the nerve occurs in the petrous part of the temporal bone, i.e. before the branch to the stapedius muscle is given off. Stapedius is protective against noise and so temporary damage to its nerve supply results in hyperacusis. Deafness is not a feature.

The patient often complains of pain behind the ear at the onset, marked unilateral facial weakness and sometimes loss of taste.

Ptosis does not occur. In fact, the opposite occurs; the eye may not close, leading to chemosis and ulceration.

1.39 Acute myocardial infarction **Answers: A B C D E**

Myocardial infarction may present with the characteristic features of severe crushing central chest pain, palpitations and nausea; but often, particularly in elderly people, symptoms are less specific or even absent. Patients presenting with injury from a fall must have the cause of the fall looked at; it may be due to an arrhythmia caused by myocardial infarction. Myocardial infarction may precipitate an acute confusional state, particularly in elderly people. In diabetic patients, a myocardial infarction may precipitate hyperglycaemia or even be silent.

Peri- or post-operative infarction may pass unnoticed until oliguria is detected. Although post-operative oliguria has many causes, for example, blood loss or dehydration, it is worth remembering that a myocardial infarction may produce a fall in cardiac output and hence oliguria.

1.40 Finger clubbing **Answers: A E**

All cyanotic congenital heart disease can cause finger clubbing; for example, transposition of the great vessels and Fallot's tetralogy. The important point is that there must be a right to left shunt. An ASD and small VSD (for example, maladie de Roger) do not produce cyanosis unless complicated by Eisenmenger's syndrome which is not mentioned in the question. Rheumatic fever does not cause clubbing but remember that subacute bacterial endocarditis can.

1.41 Cardiac arrest **Answers: B C**

Many surveys of cardiopulmonary resuscitation have shown that most junior doctors are unsafe! Recently medical schools and hospitals have improved their requirements for CPR training. Numerous questions have been set for the MRCP and OSCE examinations.

The most common cause of a cardiac arrest is ventricular fibrillation. The single lifesaving treatment is DC cardioversion and the earlier this is given the better the chance of survival. If a delay is likely, airway management and cardiac massage must be started until defibrillation is possible. Cardiac massage involves sternal compression to 1.5–2 inches at a rate of 15 compressions to 2 ventilation whether one or two people are present. Note that this is a change from the previous guidelines of 5 compressions to 1 breath if one rescuer was present. (The guidelines changed in 2001.)

The other types of cardiac arrest are asystole where QRS complexes are absent and electromechanical dissociation, i.e. the electrical activity of the heart is no longer accompanied by mechanical activity and as a result there is no cardiac output. The important causes of EMD are:

- the four H's: hypovolaemia, hypothermia, hypocalcaemia and hypoxia
- the four T's: cardiac tamponade, pulmonary thromboembolism, tension pneumothorax, toxic/therapeutic disturbances

Calcium chloride, therefore, is recommended in the management of electromechanical dissociation but not asystole. Asystole is difficult to treat. In the European protocol DC cardioversion is recommended in cases where ventricular fibrillation cannot be excluded; Atropine is given; which blocks the inhibitory effect of the vagus nerve. If QRS complexes then appear, pacing is necessary. The prognosis is poor.

1.42 Autoantibodies **Answers: B C D**

- Liver disease
  Primary biliary cirrhosis – anti-mitochondrial antibody and antinuclear factor (also raised IgM) Chronic active hepatitis - anti-smooth muscle antibody (also raised IgG)
  Alcoholic liver disease - no specific antibodies but raised IgA
- Connective tissue disease
  SLE – anti DS DNA (anti double-stranded DNA is highly specific for SLE)
  Anti-Sm (note this is not the same as anti smooth muscle antibody– Sm refers to Smith, the person who discovered the antibody)
  Anti-Ro – associated with heart block in neonates whose mothers have this antibody)
  Anti-La
- Systemic sclerosis
  Anti-Scl 70
  Anti-centromere in the CREST variant
- Polymyositis
  Anti-Jo
- Sjögren's
  Rheumatoid factor
  Anti-Ro
  Anti-La
- Rheumatoid arthritis
  Rheumatoid factor (This is IgM antibody against the Fc portion of IgG. It is not specific for rheumatoid (Rh) arthritis; 30% of patients with SLE and 90% of patients with Sjögren's have Rh factor. It also occurs in sarcoid and any condition that stimulates IgG production. Although the Rh factor titre correlates with disease activity, some patients with Rh arthritis never develop the antibody).

1.43 Chronic obstructive pulmonary disease **Answers: A B**

- Chronic obstructive pulmonary disease.
  This term is used to describe chronic bronchitis, emphysema and the spectrum that exists between them. Most people with COAD have a mixture of the two conditions.
- Chronic bronchitis
  The definition is clinical. The essential feature is a cough productive of sputum for three months of the year, for two or more consecutive years.

Pathology – there is mucus gland hypertrophy and the bronchial walls become inflamed; they undergo squamous metaplasia and fibrous changes.

Clinical features include dyspnoea and a productive cough. On examination the patient breathes with pursed lips, the chest is hyper-inflated, the crico-sternal distance is reduced and accessory muscles of respiration may be in use. The term **blue bloater** describes a patient who hypoventilates and retains carbon dioxide. Stimulation of ventilation depends on the hypoxic drive and so oxygen must be used with care. Consequences of hypoxia include:

- cyanosis (hence the term blue)
- polycythaemia because of hypoxic stimulation of erythropoietin production by the kidney (in fact, venesection may be of benefit)
- changes to pulmonary blood vessels resulting in pulmonary hypertension and cor pulmonale.

The **pink puffer** patient is less hypoxic and the patient hyperventilates in an attempt to correct poor gaseous exchange. Such patients often tolerate > 24% oxygen. It used to be thought that a blue bloater had chronic bronchitis and the pink puffer had emphysema, but post-mortem studies have not supported this. Obese patients with COAD are more likely to develop the blue bloater type of picture as obesity increases the risk of hypoventilation. Use the terms with care – some examiners like using them, but others dislike it.

- Management of acute attack
  (1) ABC – management of the airway, breathing and circulation
  (2) IV access and send blood for FBC, U&Es, blood cultures
  (3) Arterial blood gases
  (4) Controlled oxygen, i.e. 24% oxygen increased if PCO_2 allows

(5) Steroids – IV hydrocortisone or oral prednisolone
(6) Antibiotics – infected exacerbations are most likely to be due to *Haemophilus influenzae* and are treated with amoxicillin or trimethoprim or IV antibiotics if indicated
(7) Beta2-agonists (e.g. salbutamol) given as nebuliser. Anticholinergics (e.g. pratropium bromide) can also be given
(8) Physiotherapy to expel secretions
(9) Consider respiratory stimulants, such as doxapram
(10) Nasal ventilation or intubation and ventilation if clinically indicated.

- Long-term management
  (1) Stop smoking
  (2) Drugs, for example inhaled beta2 stimulants, anticholinergics, steroids
  (3) Home oxygen – this should be considered for patients with severe symptoms. There have been two major trials which show that 2 l/min of oxygen to maintain an oxygen saturation of >90% for 15 hours per day improves the symptoms. An increase to 19 hours maximum per day actually decreases mortality. Patients must have stopped smoking.
  (4) Yearly flu vaccine (provided there are no contraindications).

1.44 Rib fracture **Answers: A B C E**

Spontaneous rib fractures may occur in the absence of trauma when there is an abnormality of the rib. This may be due to osteoporosis, primary lung tumour or metastatic disease. Tumours that spread to bone include breast, lung, thyroid, kidney and prostate. Trauma may obviously cause a rib fracture but coughing, especially in elderly people, may be sufficient to cause several fractures. A rib fracture may cause a pneumothorax but not vice versa.

1.45 Rapid respiration **Answers: A B D E**

The cerebral cortex influences the respiratory rate; for example, anxiety increases the respiratory rate via increased sympathetic nervous activity. The respiratory centre in the pons responds to decreases in pH, increased H^+, increased PCO_2 and decreased PO_2 by increasing the respiratory rate. Drugs such as doxapram and aspirin in overdose can also stimulate the respiratory centre, whereas drugs such as opiates and sedatives cause hypoventilation. The pons is also influenced by peripheral chemoreceptors.

In diabetic ketoacidosis it is not the glucose level itself but the fall in pH that stimulates respiration. In uncomplicated hypoglycaemia there is no change in pH.

1.46 Pleural effusion **Answers: A B D E**

Causes of a pleural effusion can be classified according to the size of the effusion or the protein content, for example:

- Size
  Large
    neoplastic especially lung, breast, mesothelioma infection, e.g. TB
    trauma
  Moderate
    pneumonia
    heart failure
  Small
    pulmonary embolism
    pneumonia
    heart failure
    pancreatitis
    subphrenic abscess
    connective tissue disease

- Protein content
  Transudate (protein <30 g/l)
    heart failure
    liver cirrhosis
    nephrotic syndrome
    Meigs' syndrome
  Exudate (protein >30 g/l)
    malignancy (may be blood-stained)
    infection
    pulmonary embolism
    trauma
    rheumatoid arthritis – glucose content very low, rheumatoid factor high; C3, C4 (complement components) present
    subphrenic abscess (this is most common on the left side)
    pancreatitis (high amylase levels in the effusion)

Retroperitoneal fibrosis does not cause a pleural effusion.

1.47 Pupil dilatation **Answer: A**

Parasympathetic nerve fibres and fibres from the convergence centre pass via the third nerve to the pupil, resulting in pupil constriction. Sympathetic nerve stimulation causes pupil dilation. The pupil becomes smaller with age. Item C really did feature in a previous paper.

1.48 Spontaneous pneumothorax **Answers: A C**

Spontaneous pneumothorax is the sudden entry of air into a pleural space (i.e. the space between the visceral and the parietal pleura) and the subsequent collapse of the underlying lung. It occurs six times more commonly in men than in women. Symptoms range from mild pleuritic chest pain to respiratory compromise.

Investigations include a chest X-ray (NB if a tension pneumothorax is suspected this should be treated immediately even before a chest X-ray is requested). The chest X-ray confirms the diagnosis, demonstrates the presence of significant fluid levels and is used to assess the degree of collapse.

- Small pneumothorax: a rim of air is present around the lung
- Moderate sized pneumothorax: collapse halfway to the heart border
- Complete pneumothorax: airless lung separated from the diaphragm

Treatment depends on the individual patient and varies according to symptoms, the degree of collapse and whether there is underlying lung disease or bleeding. Patients should be admitted if the pneumothorax is the result of trauma or if there is underlying lung disease. Patients should also be admitted if they are symptomatic, i.e. pain is persisting or increasing or there is shortness of breath on slow walking. Patients should also be admitted if the X-ray shows a complete collapse or a fluid level is present in the costophrenic angle.

Aspiration is easy to perform. It causes minimal discomfort to the patient. Consequently, it has become a more popular treatment than intercostal tube insertion in recent years. In fact, the British Thoracic Society now recommends aspiration as the treatment of choice even in a 100% pneumothorax, i.e. complete collapse of the lung. If aspiration is not successful then intercostal drainage tube insertion is required. For guidance of chest drain insertion see question 2.12 Paper 2.

The reabsorption rate after a pneumothorax that is not treated is 1.25%/day – so a total pneumothorax would take 80 days!

1.49 Sarcoidosis **Answers: A B C D E**

Sarcoidosis is a multisystem disorder. Abnormal blood investigations include a cytopenia, occasionally eosinophilia, raised ACE, raised ESR and hypercalcaemia.

Respiratory system abnormalities are manifested by:

- chest X-ray changes, e.g. upper/mid zone fibrosis; bilateral hilar lymphadenopathy
- decreased lung volumes
- reduced diffusing capacity (KCO); normal FEV_1/ FVC ratio
- blood gases may show mild hypoxia
- gallium 67 lung scan shows increased uptake
- bronchoscopy and transbronchial biopsies or lymph node biopsies show non-caseating granulomas.

1.50 Urinary tract infection **Answers: A B C**

This is a very common question. It is designed to illustrate the non-specific, often vague symptoms that an infection may produce in elderly people, but also to warn that some symptoms are more sinister and need to be investigated thoroughly.

Any infection can produce an acute confusional state, especially in elderly people. Urinary frequency, urgency and incontinence are common symptoms, as is haematuria, but not enough to cause anaemia that should be investigated. Wandering at night is a feature of dementia.

1.51 Porto-systemic encephalography **Answers: A C D E**

Liver cirrhosis causes portal hypertension and this high pressure in the portal system opens up anastomoses with the systemic circulation. Normally toxic substances absorbed from the gut are carried in the portal circulation and broken down by the liver but now these reach the systemic circulation via the anastomoses and hence act on the brain to cause encephalopathy.

Electrolyte abnormalities and drugs that provoke them, for example diuretics, worsen encephalopathy. The brain is also exquisitely sensitive to the effects of drugs acting on the CNS, for example, opiates, benzodiazepines, which are normally metabolised by the liver.

Patients are at risk of developing oesophageal varices and consequently GI bleed. The proteins from the blood are not broken down by the liver in the normal way and these nitrogenous products are also toxic to the brain.

Bacteria in the bowel also produce nitrogenous products and if these are allowed to accumulate, for example, due to constipation, encephalopathy may be precipitated. Treatment involves correcting the underlying cause, i.e. stopping offending drugs, correcting electrolyte disturbances, and lactulose and enemas to clear the bowel. Oral neomycin used to be used to sterilise the gut, but it was found that it encouraged growth of harmful nitrogen-metabolising bacteria at the expense of useful sugar-fermenting bacteria.

General supportive care – prevention of GI bleed with attention to position to prevent aspiration, pressure sores, state of hydration, etc. – are all important in management.

1.52 Arterial blood pressure **Answers: B C D E**

This is a difficult but important question. Normally the systolic BP falls slightly on standing (<20 mmHg) and the diastolic rises slightly (>10 mmHg). A fall in systolic BP >20 mmHg or a diastolic fall ≥10 mmHg (remember the diastolic normally rises) is, by definition, postural hypotension and occurs with hypovolaemia and conditions producing autonomic dysfunction, such as diabetes mellitus, Guillain-Barré, and Shy-Drager syndromes.

The heart rate rises on standing and on exercise and these are also useful tests of autonomic function. Exercise also increases the arterial blood pressure but in the long term regular exercise lowers the blood pressure and pulse rate. There is a diurnal variation in the blood pressure – it is higher during the day.

Up to 10 mmHg difference between the right and left brachial pressures is normal. Any more than this is suggestive of aortic dissection, or if the blood pressure is elevated, coarctation of the aorta, with a stenosis proximal to the origin of the left subclavian artery.

When a small cuff is used a higher pressure is required to occlude the artery and hence the BP reading is falsely high.

1.53 Collapsing pulse **Answers: A B E**

A large volume pulse with a brisk rise and fall is known as a collapsing pulse. It is found in high cardiac output states, for example, anaemia, thyrotoxicosis, fever, aortic regurgitation and patent ductus arteriosus.

Cardiac output = stroke volume x heart rate, so if the heart rate falls the stroke volume increases to maintain the cardiac output. Bradycardia therefore causes a large volume pulse but it is not collapsing in nature. Mitral stenosis causes a reduction in cardiac output and is associated with a low volume pulse.

1.54 Mortality rates **Answers: A E**

- The **maternal mortality rate** is the number of deaths of mothers attributable to pregnancy or delivery divided by the number of births.
- The **infant mortality rate** is the number of deaths in the first year of life divided by the number of live births. It is expressed per thousand live births.
- The **neonatal mortality rate** is the number of deaths in the first four weeks of life divided by the number of live births. It is also expressed per thousand live births.
- The **perinatal mortality rate** is the number of stillbirths and deaths in the first week of life, divided by the total number of births (i.e. live and dead). It is quoted per thousand births.
- The **stillbirth rate** is the number of stillbirths divided by the total number of births (both live and stillbirth). A stillbirth is a baby born dead after 28 weeks' gestation.

1.55 Infectious diseases **Answers: A B E**

In 1992 the *Haemophilus influenzae B* vaccine (Hib) was introduced. Since then haemophilus influenza meningitis, epiglottitis and other serious infections with this organism have virtually disappeared from paediatric wards.

In 1994, measles, mumps and rubella vaccination was administered to prevent the predicted epidemic of measles in schoolchildren. The immunisation covered over 8 million children and a reduction in the number of cases of measles occurred. However in the late 1990s a link between MMR and autism was suggested. This link has never been proven and many studies have been performed which do not confirm the link. However parents have become so concerned that many have chosen not to have their children vaccinated and in 2001 several cases of measles in school children were confirmed.

Smallpox was declared to have been eradicated from the world in 1980 by the World Health Organisation. The last naturally occurring case of smallpox was in Somalia in 1977. The last epidemic of smallpox in London was at the end of the 19th century.

Influenza A viruses are antigenically labile due to changes in the surface antigen haemagglutinin (H) and neuraminidase (N). Minor changes (so called antigenic drift) occur from season to season. Major changes (i.e. antigenic shift) occur due to acquisition of a new haemagglutinin.

Influenza B may undergo minor changes (less frequently than influenza A) and does not undergo major changes.

1.56 Immunisation **Answers: B C E**

The spread of infectious disease may be reduced by social factors; for example, improvement in living conditions, better sanitation, hygiene, knowledge of spread of infections, laws governing food preparation and storage. These have had a major impact on reducing the incidence of TB, typhoid and cholera. TB spreads more rapidly where there is overcrowding, poor nutrition and poverty. Cholera is spread by water contamination and typhoid is spread by food contamination.

Vaccination is largely responsible for the decline in mortality from measles, whooping cough and diphtheria.

1.57 Inhaled steroids **Answers: B C E**

This is a difficult question and is more likely to come up as a single item rather than as a whole question.

Inhaled steroids may be low dose or high dose. There is concern regarding the safety of the latter. High dose inhaled steroids can cause adrenal suppression but this is minimal. Cushing's syndrome and cataracts are not caused by inhaled steroids even at the highest doses.

Oral candidiasis and possible laryngeal myopathy are caused by low dose inhaled steroids and are responsible for the hoarse voice often experienced by patients.

Dysphagia caused by oesophageal candidiasis can occur with the higher dose of inhaled steroids.

1.58 Polyuria **Answers: A B D**

This is a very common question. It refers to an increase in the amount of urine produced, irrespective of frequency of micturition.

ADH regulates the amount of water excretion depending on plasma osmolarity. ADH acts on the distal convoluted tubule making it permeable to water and hence promoting water reabsorption. ADH deficiency or end organ resistance to its effects will produce polyuria, for example, diabetes insipidus (cranial and nephrogenic).

The solute load through the renal tubules also determines water excretion. In diabetes mellitus there is an increased glucose load. The excess glucose inside the tubules cannot be reabsorbed (the tubular maximum for absorption has been exceeded) and the glucose is excreted in the urine. Water is retained with the glucose inside the tubules to maintain iso-osmolarity and so excess water is excreted as well as glucose. This results in polyuria and polydipsia, typical symptoms of diabetes mellitus.

Chronic hypokalaemia and hypercalcaemia damage the renal tubules producing resistance to ADH and hence polyuria.

In chronic renal failure, tubular dysfunction may result in polyuria.

An epileptic fit may cause urinary incontinence, but not polyuria.

Psychogenic causes should also be remembered, for example compulsive water drinking, which is more common in schizophrenics.

You may be asked about SVT – the answer to this is true because atrial arrhythmias stimulate atrial natriuretic peptide that causes a diuresis.

1.59 Systolic murmurs **Answers: B C D**

In general, systolic murmurs are mid or late systolic, whereas diastolic murmurs are early or mid diastolic. Aortic stenosis and pulmonary stenosis produce ejection mid systolic murmurs. Mitral valve prolapse usually produces a late systolic murmur best heard at the apex. Other causes of a late systolic murmur include coarctation of the aorta and HOCM. The murmur of HOCM is louder on squatting and standing.

The murmur of a VSD is best heard at the left sternal edge. Note that a very small VSD may produce a short murmur because contraction of the ventricle closes the defect early in systole.

The ejection systolic murmur heard with an ASD
pulmonary murmur rather than the ASD itself.

1.60 Leucocytes in urine **An**

Leucocytes in the urine occur with:

- a bacterial or chemical cystitis
- urethritis
- prostatitis
- pyelitis
- TB infection of the renal tract
- analgesic nephropathy
- renal stones

MULTIPLE CHOICE QUESTION PAPER 2

60 questions: time allowed 2½ hours
Mark your answers with a tick (True) or a cross (False) in the box provided. Leave the box blank for 'Don't know'. Do not look at the answers until you have completed the whole question paper.

2.1 Hypoglycaemia may be caused by

❑ A diabetic keto-acidosis
❑ B aspirin
❑ C alcohol
❑ D carcinoid
❑ E sepsis

2.2 Acute stroke and transient ischaemia attacks

❑ A a transient ischaemic attack often resolves within 48 hours
❑ B all patients with a stroke should have a CT scan or an MRI
❑ C all patients with a stroke should have an echo cardiogram
❑ D all patients with a stroke should have an ECG
❑ E all patients with a stroke should have a carotid duplex study

2.3 Intracranial haemorrhage

❑ A cerebellar haemorrhage requires neurosurgical referral
❑ B 10% of CT scans appear normal in the presence of a subarachnoid haemorrhage
❑ C subdural haemorrhage is usually venous in nature
❑ D extradural haemorrhage has a bi-concave or lentiform appearance
❑ E intra-cerebral haemorrhage is often due to hypertension

2.4 Status epilepticus is

❑ A a continuous generalised tonic clonic seizure
❑ B any seizure lasting more than 3 minutes
❑ C more than two discrete seizures with incomplete recovery between them
❑ D new onset epilepsy
❑ E fits occurring despite treatment

2.5 Activated charcoal reduces drug absorption of

- ❑ A ferrous sulphate
- ❑ B lithium
- ❑ C phenytoin
- ❑ D digoxin
- ❑ E aspirin

2.6 Causes of a resting tremor include

- ❑ A Parkinson's disease
- ❑ B anxiety
- ❑ C cerebellar disorders
- ❑ D alcohol withdrawal
- ❑ E hypo-thyroidism

2.7 A man of 25 years has a swollen painful knee, a prolonged partial thromboplastin time and a normal prothrombin time. The differential diagnosis includes

- ❑ A temporal arteritis
- ❑ B Christmas disease
- ❑ C haemophilia A
- ❑ D factor VII deficiency
- ❑ E von Willebrand's disease

2.8 Randomised controlled clinical trials

- ❑ A are the only convincing method of demonstrating efficacy of a drug
- ❑ B require a cross-over period
- ❑ C should be done retrospectively
- ❑ D are ideally double-blind
- ❑ E need approximately 100 subjects to detect a drug side effect

2.9 The following are complications of IV drug abuse:

- ❑ A endocarditis
- ❑ B tetanus
- ❑ C cerebral abscess
- ❑ D pulmonary embolism
- ❑ E hepatitis A

2.10 Sickle-cell anaemia is often associated with

❑ A defective urinary concentrating ability
❑ B increased risk of osteomyelitis
❑ C anaemia at birth
❑ D swollen painful hands in toddlers
❑ E enlarged spleen

2.11 Features consistent with a diagnosis of mitral stenosis include

❑ A a third heart sound
❑ B an opening snap just after the second heart sound
❑ C displaced apex beat
❑ D early diastolic murmur with presystolic accentuation
❑ E atrial fibrillation

2.12 Following refer to the insertion of an intercostal chest drain:

❑ A the drain tip should point upwards for a pleural effusion
❑ B the drain tip should point downwards for a pneumothorax
❑ C the use of a trocar is advised
❑ D an effusion is best drained with a long small-bore tube
❑ E the ideal position is the 7th intercostal space, mid-clavicular line

2.13 Causes of haemoptysis include

❑ A cystic fibrosis
❑ B Goodpasture's syndrome
❑ C lung fibrosis
❑ D tuberculosis
❑ E left ventricular failure

2.14 The following are contraindications to renal biopsy:

❑ A uncooperative patient
❑ B small kidneys
❑ C coagulation defect
❑ D single (non-transplanted) kidney
❑ E previous renal biopsy

2.15 The following skin conditions are associated with malignancy:

- ❑ A dermatomyositis
- ❑ B acanthosis nigricans
- ❑ C chronic eczema
- ❑ D psoriasis
- ❑ E mycosis fungoides

2.16 Spastic paraparesis

- ❑ A means that an arm and a leg are affected by an upper motor neurone lesion
- ❑ B in young women is most commonly caused by multiple sclerosis
- ❑ C when caused by degenerative disc disease has a poor outcome
- ❑ D does not usually affect joint position sense
- ❑ E often produces bladder symptoms

2.17 Sacroiliitis occurs in

- ❑ A rheumatoid arthritis
- ❑ B ankylosing spondylitis
- ❑ C ulcerative colitis
- ❑ D Reiter's syndrome
- ❑ E gout

2.18 Drug-induced diarrhoea is seen with

- ❑ A aluminium hydroxide
- ❑ B erythromycin
- ❑ C broad spectrum antibiotics
- ❑ D imipramine
- ❑ E loperamide

2.19 The following are causes of clubbing:

- ❑ A coeliac disease
- ❑ B atrial septal defect
- ❑ C cryptogenic fibrosing alveolitis
- ❑ D bronchiectasis
- ❑ E COAD

2.20 Increased skin pigmentation occurs with

- ❑ A hypopituitarism
- ❑ B haemochromatosis
- ❑ C chronic renal failure
- ❑ D varicose eczema
- ❑ E vitiligo

2.21 Regarding hepatitis A infection:

- ❑ A 10% of patients develop liver cirrhosis
- ❑ B anorexia is a prominent early symptom
- ❑ C it may be spread by faecal contamination
- ❑ D it may be fatal
- ❑ E it always requires admission to an isolation unit

2.22 Severe acute abdominal pain is a feature of

- ❑ A coeliac disease
- ❑ B acute intermittent porphyria
- ❑ C lower lobe pneumonia
- ❑ D diabetic keto-acidosis
- ❑ E infection with herpes zoster at T10

2.23 Difficulty swallowing can occur as a result of the following conditions:

- ❑ A oesophageal reflux
- ❑ B carcinoma of the stomach
- ❑ C motor neurone disease
- ❑ D depression
- ❑ E recurrent laryngeal nerve palsy

2.24 Regarding lung cancer

- ❑ A smokers tend to develop adenocarcinoma
- ❑ B vocal cord palsy indicates inoperability
- ❑ C tumours are more easily resected if close to the hilum
- ❑ D small cell carcinoma can be treated by chemotherapy
- ❑ E the brain is a common site for metastases

2.25 Proximal muscle weakness is a well recognised feature of

- ❑ A osteoporosis
- ❑ B thyrotoxicosis
- ❑ C corticosteroid therapy
- ❑ D muscular dystrophy
- ❑ E diabetes mellitus

2.26 The following are true of renal amyloid:

- ❑ A it produces large kidneys
- ❑ B prognosis is poor
- ❑ C staining with Congo red is characteristic
- ❑ D it may present with chronic renal failure
- ❑ E it may be caused by chronic infection

2.27 The following skin lesions are correctly paired with the disease stated:

❑	A	pyoderma gangrenosum	diabetes mellitus
❑	B	erythema multiforme	rheumatic fever
❑	C	rose spots	typhoid fever
❑	D	skin ulcers	sickle-cell anaemia
❑	E	erythema nodosum	ulcerative colitis

2.28 Increased sweating is a recognised feature of

- ❑ A diabetic keto-acidosis
- ❑ B phaeochromocytoma
- ❑ C left ventricular failure
- ❑ D cystic fibrosis
- ❑ E acromegaly

2.29 Herpes simplex virus may

- ❑ A produce a severe generalised eruption in children with eczema
- ❑ B cause corneal lesions
- ❑ C cause encephalitis
- ❑ D be sensitive to acyclovir
- ❑ E result in post-herpetic neuralgia

2.30 Gynaecomastia is a feature of

❑ A lung cancer
❑ B old age
❑ C obesity
❑ D hypothyroidism
❑ E hypercholesterolaemia

2.31 An acute asthmatic attack may be precipitated by

❑ A exercise
❑ B selective beta1-receptor blocking drugs
❑ C prednisolone
❑ D ibuprofen
❑ E adrenaline

2.32 Causes of generalised lymphadenopathy include

❑ A sarcoid
❑ B lymphoma
❑ C tuberculosis
❑ D chronic lymphocytic lymphoma
❑ E lymphoedema

2.33 The following are causes of diastolic murmurs:

❑ A Austin Flint murmur
❑ B Graham Steell murmur
❑ C mitral valve prolapse
❑ D mitral regurgitation
❑ E pulmonary regurgitation

2.34 Causes of a large tongue include

❑ A vitamin B12 deficiency
❑ B acromegaly
❑ C Down's syndrome
❑ D amyloid
❑ E syphilis

2.35 Dementia

❑ A is termed presenile if it occurs before the age of 75
❑ B is always progressive
❑ C may be caused by head injury
❑ D can be diagnosed by a mini mental test score of 6
❑ E causes a reversal of the sleep-wake cycle

2.36 The following refer to pulmonary tuberculosis:

❑ A it is unlikely if the chest X-ray is normal
❑ B a Heaf test of >10 mm is suggestive
❑ C *Mycobacterium bacillus* can be grown from blood culture
❑ D the BCG vaccine is >90% protective for life
❑ E rifampicin causes optic neuropathy

2.37 Dark urine occurs with

❑ A beetroot consumption
❑ B heavy proteinuria
❑ C porphyria
❑ D malaria
❑ E Gilbert's syndrome

2.38 Interferon may be of benefit in the following:

❑ A hepatitis A
❑ B chronic hepatitis B
❑ C chronic hepatitis C
❑ D multiple sclerosis
❑ E depression

2.39 The following may provoke an epileptic seizure:

❑ A flashing lights
❑ B illness
❑ C head injury
❑ D family argument
❑ E anticonvulsants

2.40 The management of osteoporosis includes

- ❑ A avoiding exercise whenever possible
- ❑ B stopping smoking
- ❑ C increasing dietary calcium
- ❑ D hormone replacement therapy
- ❑ E avoiding travel by aeroplane

2.41 The following drugs have been shown to decrease mortality after myocardial infarction:

- ❑ A aspirin
- ❑ B beta-blockers
- ❑ C rTPA
- ❑ D ACE inhibitors
- ❑ E oral magnesium

2.42 Hypothyroidism may cause

- ❑ A dementia
- ❑ B hypothermia
- ❑ C hirsutism
- ❑ D coma
- ❑ E pretibial myxoedema

2.43 Ulceration inside the mouth occurs in

- ❑ A Behçet's syndrome
- ❑ B ulcerative colitis
- ❑ C SLE
- ❑ D pemphigus vulgaris
- ❑ E stress

2.44 Risk factors for large bowel malignancy include

- ❑ A constipation
- ❑ B family history
- ❑ C ulcerative colitis
- ❑ D Crohn's disease
- ❑ E diverticular disease

2.45 The following are features of a cerebellopontine angle tumour:

- ❑ A facial weakness
- ❑ B facial numbness
- ❑ C deafness
- ❑ D ataxia
- ❑ E optic atrophy

2.46 The following suggest a median nerve injury:

- ❑ A inability to oppose the thumb to the little finger
- ❑ B inability to adduct the thumb
- ❑ C sensory loss over the medial one and a half fingers
- ❑ D pain in the upper arm
- ❑ E tingling in the forearm

2.47 In elderly people

- ❑ A a UTI may cause coma
- ❑ B part III accommodation is only for people who are continent
- ❑ C Erythema ab igne may indicate hypothyroidism
- ❑ D cardiopulmonary resuscitation should not be performed on patients over the age of 85
- ❑ E a haemoglobin level of 10 is within the normal range

2.48 Causes of an eosinophilia include

- ❑ A asthma
- ❑ B Hodgkin's lymphoma
- ❑ C psoriasis
- ❑ D eczema
- ❑ E rheumatoid arthritis

2.49 A pleural effusion is often associated with

- ❑ A oesophageal rupture
- ❑ B COAD
- ❑ C sarcoid
- ❑ D liver cirrhosis
- ❑ E diabetic keto-acidosis

2.50 Regarding left ventricular failure:

- ❑ A frusemide is used acutely for its immediate diuretic effect
- ❑ B ACE inhibitors decrease mortality and morbidity
- ❑ C a change in heart size on chest radiograph will be visible within 24 hours of treatment for the acute attack
- ❑ D a gallop rhythm indicates inadequate treatment
- ❑ E pulsus alternans indicates a poor prognosis

2.51 The following can produce symptoms suggestive of schizophrenia:

- ❑ A amphetamine addiction
- ❑ B pregnancy
- ❑ C opiate abuse
- ❑ D temporal lobe epilepsy
- ❑ E hypoglycaemia

2.52 Hirsutism is caused by

- ❑ A polycystic ovarian syndrome
- ❑ B congenital adrenal hyperplasia
- ❑ C porphyria cutanea tarda
- ❑ D acromegaly
- ❑ E thyrotoxicosis

2.53 Abnormal speech is a recognised feature of

- ❑ A ill-fitting dentures
- ❑ B Parkinson's disease
- ❑ C motor neurone disease
- ❑ D multiple sclerosis
- ❑ E hypoglossal nerve damage

2.54 Ulcerative colitis is associated with

- ❑ A dermatitis herpetiformis
- ❑ B erythema nodosum
- ❑ C liver cirrhosis
- ❑ D arthritis
- ❑ E sclerosing cholangitis

2.55 The following refer to splitting of the second heart sound:

- ❑ A reversed splitting occurs in left bundle branch block
- ❑ B fixed splitting occurs only in an atrial septal defect
- ❑ C wide splitting occurs in pulmonary stenosis
- ❑ D it is normal to hear splitting in the mitral area
- ❑ E the aortic second sound is louder in aortic stenosis

2.56 The following infectious diseases are transmitted by ticks:

- ❑ A malaria
- ❑ B dengue fever
- ❑ C Chagas disease
- ❑ D Lyme disease
- ❑ E yellow fever

2.57 The following are true:

- ❑ A in a normal distribution, the mean, mode, and median may be but are not always the same
- ❑ B the median is the most frequently occurring value
- ❑ C the standard deviation refers to a measure of the spread of a normally distributed population
- ❑ D in a normal distribution, ±1 SD includes 68% of the population
- ❑ E in a normal distribution, ±3 SD includes 99% of the population

2.58 The following are true:

- ❑ A the standard error of the mean = the standard deviation divided by the square of the number of values in the sample
- ❑ B a p value of 0.005 implies statistical significance
- ❑ C a type 1 error results in a significant difference being obtained when it should not have been
- ❑ D a paired t test may be used for comparison of means for normally distributed populations only
- ❑ E the c2 test may be performed on means

2.59 Photosensitivity occurs in

- ❑ A SLE
- ❑ B amiodarone treatment
- ❑ C acute intermittent porphyria
- ❑ D pellagra
- ❑ E scurvy

2.60 Causes of chorea include

- ❑ A thyrotoxicosis
- ❑ B Huntington's chorea
- ❑ C rheumatic fever
- ❑ D pregnancy
- ❑ E cerebellar lesion

END

Go over your answers until your time is up.
Correct answers and teaching notes are overleaf.

MULTIPLE CHOICE QUESTION PAPER 2 – ANSWERS

The correct answer options for each question are given below.

2.1	B C D E	2.31	A B D
2.2	B D	2.32	A B C D
2.3	A C D E	2.33	A B E
2.4	A C	2.34	B C D
2.5	C D E	2.35	C E
2.6	A B D	2.36	A E
2.7	B C	2.37	A C D
2.8	D	2.38	B C D
2.9	A B C D	2.39	A B C D E
2.10	A B D	2.40	B C D
2.11	B E	2.41	A B C D
2.12	All false	2.42	A B D
2.13	A B D E	2.43	A D E
2.14	A B C D	2.44	A B C
2.15	A B E	2.45	A B C D
2.16	B E	2.46	A E
2.17	B C D	2.47	A B C
2.18	B C	2.48	A B D E
2.19	A C D	2.49	A D
2.20	B C D	2.50	B C D E
2.21	B C D	2.51	A B C D E
2.22	B C D E	2.52	A B C D E
2.23	B C D	2.53	A B C D E
2.24	B D E	2.54	B C D E
2.25	B C D E	2.55	A B C
2.26	A B C D E	2.56	D
2.27	A C D E	2.57	C D E
2.28	A B C E	2.58	B C D
2.29	A B C D	2.59	A B D
2.30	A B	2.60	A B C D

MCQ PAPER 2 – ANSWERS AND TEACHING NOTES

2.1 Hypoglycaemia — Answers: B C D E

Hypoglycaemia is unusual except in patients with diabetes who are prescribed hypoglycaemic drugs. Occasionally other drugs such as alcohol and aspirin may cause hypoglycaemia. Tumours such as insulinoma and carcinoid also cause hypoglycaemia. Sepsis usually causes hyperglycaemia but may also cause hypoglycaemia especially in neonates.

Glucose must be given IMMEDIATELY. If possible it should be given by mouth but where this is not possible it should be administered intravenously. The oral route is preferable and it is equally effective without the risk of tissue necrosis that may occur with intravenous administration if the needle is not properly sited within a vein.

Diabetic ketoacidosis is the result of a lack of insulin and hyperglycaemia.

2.2 Acute stroke and transcient ischaemia — Answers: B D

By definition, a transient ischaemic attack resolves within 24 hours and often within one hour. All patients with a stroke should have a CT or MRI scan, preferably within 48 hours but more urgently if there is worsening neurology. A scan is needed to differentiate infarction from haemorrhage and exclude other causes of neurology such as tumour, AVM, subarachnoid haemorrhage. The scan will also identify patients requiring urgent surgical referral.

An echocardiogram is only required if there is significant cardiac abnormality on clinical examination or if the patient is < 60 years old. Patients who are <50 years old with recurrent unexplained stroke should have a trans-oesophageal echocardiogram.

An ECG will identify arrhythmia such as atrial-fibrillation and should be performed in all patients with a stroke.

Carotid duplex studies are only necessary for a carotid territory stroke or if the territory of the stroke is uncertain.

All patients should have a full blood count, ESR, urea and creatinine and electrolytes, glucose, cholesterol and a chest X-ray. If there is an haemorrhagic stroke (blood is seen on CT/MRI) a clotting screen should be performed. If the patient has had an ischaemic stroke and is below 60 years of age a thrombophilia screen should be performed and auto-antibodies and anti-cardiolipin measurements performed.

2.3 Intracranial haemorrhage **Answers: A C D E**

The term intracranial haemorrhage means that bleeding has occurred within the brain or subarachnoid or subdural or extradural spaces.

Cerebellar haemorrhage is of great concern as there is little space within the posterior fossa and bleeding rapidly causes compression with the danger of herniation and death. Urgent neuro-surgical referral is required. A CT scan is very sensitive in detection of blood. However, up to 1% of subarachnoid haemorrhages will have normal CT scan and a lumbar puncture is required to detect the haemorrhage.

A subdural haemorrhage is usually due to a venous bleed. On a CT scan it has a crescentic appearance. An extradural haemorrhage is usually due to an arterial bleed and on a CT scan has a bi-concave or lentiform appearance.

2.4 Status epilepticus **Answers: A C**

Status epilepticus is defined as either continuous, generalised, tonic-clonic seizures or tonic-clonic seizures that are so frequent that each attack begins before the post-ictal period of the preceding one ends.

The mortality is high and it is important to control the fits as soon as possible. As with all medical emergencies management begins with ABC, i.e. airway, breathing and circulation.

Make the environment safe for the patients, e.g. using padded bed rails to keep the patient from damaging themself. When possible, place the patient in a semi-prone position with the head down, maintain airway and help prevent aspiration. If possible, during an inter-ictal period, insert an airway and administer oxygen.

Set up an intravenous line as soon as possible and send venous blood for measurement of glucose, urea and electrolytes, calcium, liver function, full blood count and clotting, and anti-convulsant blood levels.

The blood glucose should be assessed rapidly using a BM test and if the patient is hypoglycaemic 50% glucose should be administered rapidly, but do not wait for the formal blood glucose level to come back from the laboratory.

Check body temperature and blood pressure and do an ECG.

If possible get a history from an accompanying person and look for clues on the patient that might help with management such as a medic alert bracelet. The seizures should be terminated with a benzodiazepine such as lorazepam or diazepam. The patient should also be given IV Phenytoin which will help stop seizures if they are still continuing and also prevent further ones.

If seizures do not stop on this regime, the patient should be transferred to an ITU and a neurological opinion urgently sought.

2.5 Charcoal **Answers: C D E**

Activated charcoal both decreases absorption of most drugs and increases elimination by interrupting the entero-enteric and entero-hepatic circuits. It will not work with mineral acids, lithium, DDT, cyanide or ferrous sulphate.

It is by far the most effective treatment for most drugs and should be considered the treatment of choice in the first 1.5 hours after overdose, with or without gastric lavage preceding the dose. Some drugs such as tricyclic and opiates delay gastric emptying and so lavage and activated charcoal can be performed even if overdosage was up to 12 hours earlier.

2.6 Resting tremor **Answers: A B D**

The cerebellar tremor is an intention tremor and does not typically occur at rest. Causes of a resting tremor include anxiety, beta-agonist drugs, alcohol intoxication or withdrawal, thyrotoxicosis, familial tremor and basal ganglia lesions, for example, Parkinson's disease. Note that the tremor of Parkinson's is a pill rolling rest tremor which decreases on intentional movement in contrast to a cerebellar tremor.

2.7 Coagulation **Answers: B C**

The extrinsic and intrinsic pathways lead to the final common pathway; this results in thrombin production which activates fibrinogen conversion to fibrin, allowing clot formation. The extrinsic pathway involves tissue thromboplastin and Factor VII and is measured by the prothrombin time (PT time). The intrinsic pathway involves XII, XI, IX , VIII, platelet phospholipid and calcium. The final common pathway involves Factors X, V, calcium and formation of II (prothrombin). The intrinsic pathway and final common pathway is measured by the APTT (also known as the PTT and the KCCT). The conversion of fibrinogen to fibrin by thrombin is measured by the thrombin time (TT). Temporal arteritis is a vasculitis and does not affect the clotting pathway.

2.8 Randomised controlled clinical trials Answer: D

A double-blind randomised controlled trial is the ideal way of assessing efficacy of a drug. The term double-blind means that the patient and the doctor do not know whether the patient is receiving the drug or a placebo, or the drug being studied and an established drug for comparison. The study may be done in parallel or cross-over. In the latter one group of patients start on the new drug and are then swapped over to the old drug or placebo. The other group is started on the established treatment or placebo and then changed over to the drug being studied.

The more patients that are studied the better, so that the less common side effects can be picked up.

2.9 Complications of IV drug abuse Answers: A B C D

Apart from the side-effects of the drugs involved, intravenous drug abuse has numerous problems. Needle sharing transmits blood-borne viruses such as HIV, hepatitis B and hepatitis C. Hepatitis A is water borne and transmitted by the faeco-oral route.

An infected needle allows bacteria to reach the heart, in particular the valves producing endocarditis. It is theoretically possible for micro-organisms to reach the brain, causing a cerebral abscess but a right to left shunt would be required for this. Dirty needles may also allow tetanus to be introduced. Large particles injected into a vein, particularly the large femoral vein could produce a significant pulmonary embolus.

2.10 Sickle cell anaemia associations Answers: A B D

Sickle-cell anaemia does not present at birth, as fetal haemoglobin is still present. When cells sickle they block small vessels causing infarction and damage to numerous organs. For example, splenic infarction results in a small spleen. In the kidneys tubular dysfunction occurs causing a defective urinary concentrating ability. Bone infarction causes pain (painful dactylitis in toddlers) and also increases the risk of osteomyelitis. Patients who have a reduced splenic function are also at risk of overwhelming septicaemia from pneumococcus and meningococcus in particular. A chest crisis may occur, severe shunting and hypoxia caused by intra-pulmonary sickling may spread throughout the lungs, mimicking pulmonary embolism and pneumonia. Cerebral sickling causes the patient to have fits, strokes, coma, bizarre behaviour or psychosis.

If sickling occurs within the splanchnic bed the patient may develop abdominal pain with signs of peritonism and jaundice, which is known as girdle syndrome.

2.11 Mitral stenosis **Answers: B E**

The presence of a third heart sound, a displaced apex beat and an early diastolic murmur make the diagnosis of mitral stenosis unlikely.

Symptoms of mitral stenosis:

- Dyspnoea – as the left atrium hypertrophies the left atrial pressure rises. The pulmonary venous pressure then rises causing pulmonary venous hypertension. Increased venous pressure in any part of the body will produce oedema and in the lungs it is referred to as pulmonary oedema.
- Fatigue, weakness – the low cardiac output which occurs with valve stenoses gives rise to this. Development of cor pulmonale exacerbates these symptoms.
- Palpitations – atrial fibrillation occurs secondary to the enlarged left atrium.
- Emboli – atrial fibrillation increases the risk of thrombosis and pulmonary and systemic emboli.
- Dysphagia – rarely, the enlarged left atrium compresses the oesophagus to produce dysphagia.

Signs of mitral stenosis:

- Inspection – mitral facies
- Pulse – this is irregular in both rate and volume – this is the correct way to describe the pulse in atrial fibrillation.
- Precordium

  Palpation – right ventricular heave, tapping apex beat – not displaced because the ventricle is normal in size.

  Auscultation – the first heart sound is loud (the stenosed valve slams shut). A loud P2 occurs with pulmonary hypertension and an opening snap may be heard as the valve opens in diastole. If the left atrial pressure is very high, as with severe mitral stenosis, the valve may open earlier. Therefore the opening snap is heard earlier, i.e. closer to the second heart sound.

  There is a mid-diastolic, low pitched rumbling murmur best heard with the bell, just lateral to the apex beat. It is best heard in the left lateral position in expiration and is increased with exercise. Presystolic accentuation may occur if the patient is in sinus rhythm as atrial contraction forces more blood through the valve increasing the turbulence, and hence the loudness of the murmur.

2.12 Intercostal chest drain **Answers: All false**

A narrow bore intercostal chest drain is used for draining a pneumothorax and should be inserted pointing upwards. Drainage for an effusion is with a large bore drain and is inserted pointing downwards.

Insertion should be by blunt dis-section; a trocar is no longer recommended. For greatest safety the chest drain should be inserted in the triangle bounded by the apex of the axilla, the nipple (4th intercostal space in the mid-clavicular line) and the base of the scapula.

2.13 Haemoptysis **Answers: A B D E**

Haemoptysis refers to the coughing up of blood or blood-stained sputum. This will occur if there is damage to the bronchi or air spaces, or damage to the blood vessels. It is less likely to occur when damage is of the interstitial lung tissues, for example, lung fibrosis.

Diseases of the bronchi and its connections:

- primary tumours – secondary tumours tend to metastasize to the interstitium
- infection – pneumonia, lung abscess, TB
- bronchial wall damage – for example, cystic fibrosis, bronchiectasis

Lesions of the blood vessel:

- lumen – for example, pulmonary embolus
- wall – vasculitis, for example, Goodpasture's, Wegener's and Churg-Strauss syndromes.

Raised pulmonary venous pressure, for example, mitral stenosis, left ventricular failure makes the vessels more liable to rupture and bleed.

2.14 Renal biopsy **Answers: A B C D**

Consent is required for all invasive procedures. If a patient will not consent or is uncooperative, no invasive procedure should be performed.

Most renal biopsies are performed to determine the underlying cause of renal failure. If the kidneys are small and shrunken this implies the disease process has already gone too far and determining a diagnosis at this stage is too late. Also, small kidneys are difficult to biopsy and histology is difficult to interpret.

A single post-transplant kidney may be biopsied when rejection appears to be occurring. However, if a non-transplant patient has only one kidney, this should not be biopsied as 1 in 400 patients have profuse post-biopsy haemorrhage requiring occlusion of the bleeding vessel at angiography or even nephrectomy.

Repeated renal biopsies are often necessary to determine rejection or to monitor response to treatment.

2.15 Skin conditions associated with malignancy **Answers: A B E**

Dermatomyositis occurs with increased incidence in carcinoma of the bronchus and ovaries. A purplish discoloration around the eyelids and knuckles is characteristic.

Acanthosis nigricans is a dark velvety rash especially under the axilla. It is associated with gastric and other intra-abdominal malignancy. Ninety per cent of patients with acanthosis nigricans have a malignancy.

Mycosis fungoides is a T-cell lymphoma initially confined to the skin.
Erythema gyratum repens consists of concentric erythematous rings over the whole body. It is associated with carcinoma of the bronchus.

Necrolytic migratory erythema is associated with glucagonoma.

Migrating thrombophlebitis is associated with carcinoma of the pancreas.
Ichthyosis is skin thickening associated with lymphoma.

Eczema and psoriasis are not associated with malignancy. Psoriasis can be treated with methotrexate which increases the risk of haemopoietic malignancy, but the question refers to the skin condition and not to the treatment.

2.16 Spastic paraparesis **Answers: B E**

Spastic paraparesis refers to the upper motor neurone weakness of both legs.

In young women, demyelination (for example, multiple sclerosis) is the most likely cause but other important causes include:

- cord compression – this needs to be above the level of L1: the cord ends here and lesions below it will not produce a spastic paraparesis. Causes include degenerative disc disease, disc prolapse and tumours. Degenerative disc disease/disc prolapse is amenable to surgery and usually produces excellent results: recovery may be full.
- motor neurone disease
- birth injury
- sub-acute combined degeneration of the cord
- syringomyelia
- para-sagittal meningioma
- treponemal disease, generalized paralysis of the insane (GPI), taboparesis
- hereditary, for example, Friedreich's ataxia

Option D is difficult. Usually a spastic paraparesis will produce sensory and motor changes and joint position sense is often lost. There is an exception – motor neurone disease only affects motor neurones, therefore technically joint position sense is preserved.

Remember that in multiple sclerosis only the central nervous system is affected but both the motor and sensory systems can be involved. In motor neurone disease only the motor system is affected but both the central and peripheral nervous systems are involved.

2.17 Sacroiliitis **Answers: B C D**

The easiest way to remember the causes of sacroiliitis is to think of the associations and causes of the sero-negative spondarthritis *PUB CAR:*

Psoriasis
Ulcerative colitis
Behçet's disease
Crohn's disease
Ankylosing spondylitis
Reiter's disease

Note that Whipple's disease is seronegative but does not usually cause sacroiliitis.

2.18 Drug-induced diarrhoea **Answers: B C**

Increased transit time (producing constipation) is caused by:

- sympathetic nervous system stimulation
- opiate receptor stimulation, for example, codeine, loperamide
- parasympathetic nervous system inhibition, for example anticholinergics and antidepressants
- aluminium salts

Decreased transit time (producing diarrhoea) is caused by:

- parasympathetic nervous system stimulation
- sympathetic nervous system inhibition
- alteration of bacterial flora, for example antibiotic-associated diarrhoea or pseudomembranous colitis. Note that erythromycin also has a pro-kinetic effect on the gut as well as altering bacterial flora
- magnesium salts

2.19 Clubbing **Answers: A C D**

Nail clubbing only occurs when fibrosis, infective or inflammatory conditions are chronic:

- Heart
  Cyanotic congenital heart disease (atrial septal defect is not cyanotic); subacute bacterial endocarditis
- Lungs
  Infective or inflammatory: tuberculosis, bronchiectasis, lung abscess, empyema, bronchial carcinoma, mesothelioma
  Fibrotic: cryptogenic fibrosing alveolitis
  Chronic obstructive airways disease (COAD) is NOT a cause of clubbing – if it is present think of a co-existing malignancy
- Gastrointestinal
  Inflammatory bowel disease, liver cirrhosis, coeliac disease, gastrointestinal lymphoma

2.20 Skin pigmentation **Answers: B C D**

Increased skin pigmentation has many causes:

- Raised melanin – haemochromatosis; Addison's disease – stimulates increased MSH and ACTH; hyperthyroidism; renal failure – increased MSH-like hormone production.
- Haemosiderin – extravasated blood from venous ulcers can cause localised melanin production.
- Increased ACTH – ACTH also has melanocyte stimulatory hormone activity; Addison's disease; oat cell tumours of the bronchus; Cushing's disease.

Other causes of increased local pigmentation are:

- acanthosis nigricans
- systemic sclerosis
- pregnancy/OCP
- neurofibromatosis

2.21 Hepatitis A infection **Answers: B C D**

Hepatitis A virus is spread by the faeco-oral route. It has an incubation period of about two weeks. The pre-icteric period is up to 2 weeks. During this time, patients experience nausea, vomiting, anorexia, headache and malaise. During the icteric period the patient often feels better. On examination, 10% have hepatomegaly; there may also be lymphadenopathy and in some cases a rash. Rarely, fulminant hepatitis develops resulting in coma and death.

Cirrhosis does not occur. Mild cases may be managed at home.

2.22 Acute abdominal pain **Answers: B C D E**

Obvious causes of severe acute abdominal pain include infection, inflammation and perforation of abdominal organs.

Important causes include lower lobe pneumonia (the pain of which may be referred down as far as the right iliac fossa, mimicking appendicitis); diabetic ketoacidosis causing gastric stasis and ileus; thoracic *Herpes zoster*; acute intermittent porphyria.

Coeliac disease can cause abdominal distension or bloating but tends not to produce severe acute abdominal pain.

2.23 Dysphagia **Answers: B C D**

See also Paper 1, Question 1.28. Oesophageal reflux tends to produce heartburn and retrosternal pain. Unless stricture formation has occurred dysphagia is not a usual feature.

Carcinoma of the stomach, in particular of the fundus, can compress the oesophagus, producing dysphagia.

Motor neurone disease causes weakness of the pharyngeal muscles.

Depression causes a functional dysphagia.

Recurrent laryngeal nerve palsy causes dysphasia, not dysphagia.

2.24 Lung cancer **Answers: B D E**

Lung carcinoma is divided into small cell and non-small cell carcinoma:

- Small cell carcinoma
  Oat cell – this arises from endocrine cells which secrete polypeptide hormones. These are highly malignant and rapid growing but respond well to chemotherapy.

- Non-small cell carcinoma
  Squamous cell carcinoma – 40% of all lung carcinomas. Cavitates, metastasizes late.
  Large cell carcinomas – 25% of tumours; metastasizes early.
  Adenocarcinoma – 10% of tumours. Arises in scar tissue, therefore is associated with asbestosis. Proportionally more common in non-smokers, women and elderly people.
  Alveolar cell carcinoma – 1–2% of tumours. These patients produce large amounts of mucoid sputum.
  The treatment for small cell carcinoma is chemotherapy. For non-small cell carcinoma the treatment is surgery +/or chemotherapy.
  Surgery is only an option if

- the tumour is not too near the hilum
- there is no evidence of metastasis
- FEV_1 >1.5 l
- there is no vocal cord paralysis

Carcinoma of the lung metastasizes to brain, bone and liver.

2.25 Proximal muscle weakness **Answers: B C D E**

Proximal muscle weakness means weakness predominantly affecting the shoulder/pelvic girdle. It is caused by:

- Muscle disorders – for example, polymyositis, muscular dystrophy, myotonic dystrophy.
- Endocrine disorders – thyrotoxicosis, hypothyroidism, Cushing's disease.
- Metabolic disorders – osteomalacia, steroid therapy, hypokalaemia.

2.26 Renal amyloid **Answers: A B C D E**

Small kidneys are usually a feature of most chronic renal disorders, the exceptions being hydronephrosis, polycystic renal disease and renal amyloid that produce large kidneys.

Amyloidosis is a disorder of protein metabolism. It consists of protein fibrils that stain red with Congo red and show a green fluorescence in polarised light. It may be primary or secondary to chronic infection. In the secondary form serum amyloid A, which is an acute phase protein, is overproduced and becomes deposited in organs.

2.27 Skin lesions **Answers: A C D E**

Diabetes mellitus is associated with pyoderma gangrenosum and necrobiosis lipoidica. It may cause lipoatrophy or lipohypertrophy (related to insulin injection site), and certain skin infections (e.g. candidiasis) are more common in diabetics.

A previous stem referred to necrolytic migrating erythema; this is associated with a glucagonoma which can produce diabetes mellitus.

Rheumatic fever can cause erythema marginatum. Erythema multiforme is associated with herpes simplex infection (Type 1), *Mycoplasma pneumoniae,* drugs such as sulphonamides and barbiturates, Streptococcus, Yersinia, and neoplasia. In 50% of cases no cause is found. Rose spots are a macular papular rash appearing on the upper abdomen/thorax during the second week of a typhoid illness.

For causes of erythema nodosum see Paper 1, Question 1.17.

2.28 Sweating **Answers: A C E**

An increase in sympathetic nervous system activity occurs with anxiety, heart failure, pheochromocytoma and fever.

In ketoacidosis there is profound dehydration and the skin is usually dry. Excess growth hormone affects the sweat glands, causing increased sweating and greasy skin.

The trick in this question is cystic fibrosis. Everyone remembers the abnormal sweat test and therefore marks this as true, but in fact it is the amount of sodium and not the amount of sweat that is increased.

2.29 Herpes simplex virus **Answers: A B C D**

Herpes simplex is a DNA pox virus. Type 1 causes oral lesions and Type 2 causes genital lesions, but this is not absolute.

Trauma to the skin or a mucosal surface – for example, the eye, genital area or mouth – allows introduction of the virus. Primary infection of genital herpes is usually more severe than primary oral infection. The latter may be asymptomatic, or may cause marked localised pain, ulceration and systemic illness.

The virus lies dormant in the dorsal root ganglion and may periodically reactivate. In genital herpes, recurrences are inevitable.

People at risk of severe infection include:

- immunocompromised inpatients
- neonates (Caesarian section should be performed)
- atopic individuals (even if eczema is not in an active phase, eczema herpeticum may occur, post-herpetic neuralgia refers to the pain in the dermatome affected by shingles (*Herpes zoster* and not *Herpes simplex*).

2.30 Gynaecomastia **Answers: A B**

Causes of gynaecomastia include:

- Physiological – neonatal, puberty, old age
- Endocrine – hyperthyroidism
- Metabolic – starvation and refeeding, oestrogen excess and testosterone deficiency
- Tumours – human chorionic gonadotrophin (HCG) producing lung and testicular tumours. Note therefore that testicular tumours can produce gynaecomastia by production of oestrogen or HCG

- Drugs – see Paper 1, Question 1.15

Obesity causes an increase in breast size due to fat deposition, but not true breast tissue development.

2.31 Acute asthma **Answers: A B D**

Bronchial hyper-responsiveness is thought to be responsible for symptoms in asthma. The airways are thought to be more sensitive to cold air and irritants, such as dust. The immediate effect of exercise is bronchodilation followed by bronchoconstriction, the latter being exaggerated in asthmatic patients. Patients often complain that they are extremely short of breath 10–15 minutes after stopping exercise.

Airway tone is normally under the influence of the following:

- sympathetic nerve system which dilates the airways via beta2-receptor stimulation
- parasympathetic nerve stimulation by the vagus nerve induces bronchial constriction
- cyclic AMP activation
- numerous other receptors, for example, adenosine receptors

Although it is obvious that beta2-receptor blocking drugs will cause bronchial constriction, it must also be appreciated that even highly selective beta1-receptor blocking drugs have the potential to cause a fatal asthmatic attack and are contraindicated.

Drugs potentiating the sympathetic nervous system, such as adrenaline, will cause bronchial dilation and until quite recently adrenaline was first-line treatment for an asthmatic attack. Newer treatments include beta2-receptor stimulation by drugs such as salbutamol and the longer acting salmeterol.

Drugs inhibiting the parasympathetic nervous system include ipratropium bromide which by its anticholinergic effect helps to relax the airways. The theophylline group of drugs are phosphodiesterase inhibitors which help to potentiate the effect of cyclic AMP and this also results in airway dilatation.

Bronchoconstriction is not the only problem during an acute asthmatic attack; in addition there is marked inflammation and steroids, such as prednisolone, have considerable benefit but take several hours to work.

However, drugs such as non-steroidal anti-inflammatories (NSAIDs), act by diverting the precursors from the cyclooxygenase to the lipoxygenase pathway resulting in increased production of leukotrienes which are potent bronchoconstrictors. These drugs should therefore be avoided.

This is a very important question and frequently comes up.

2.32 Generalised lymphadenopathy **Answers: A B C D**

The causes of generalised lymphadenopathy are:

- lymphoma – lymph nodes are said to be rubbery and firm
- leukaemia – chronic lymphocytic leukaemia and acute lymphoblastic leukaemia in particular
- malignancies – the nodes tend to be very firm and asymmetrical
- infection: viral (e.g. CMV, HIV, infection, infectious mononucleosis); bacterial (e.g. TB, brucellosis); protozoa (e.g. toxoplasmosis)
- connective tissue diseases (e.g. rheumatoid arthritis, SLE)
- infiltrative/granulomatous disorders (e.g. sarcoid drugs, such as phenytoin)

Lymphoedema is caused by obstruction to lymphatic flow and does not produce a generalised lymphadenopathy.

2.33 Diastolic murmurs **Answers: A B E**

Diastolic murmurs may be divided into mid-diastolic or early diastolic. Mid-diastolic murmurs include the murmur of mitral stenosis, best heard at the apex with the patient on the left side, and accentuated on exertion. It is of low frequency and rumbling in nature.

Tricuspid stenosis is also mid-diastolic, best heard at the left sternal edge and louder on inspiration.

The Austin Flint murmur is produced when aortic regurgitation causes a jet of blood to hit the mitral valve; it is best heard at the apex.

Early diastolic murmurs – aortic regurgitation is best heard at the left sternal edge and the apex, with the patient sitting forward in held expiration. It is a blowing high-pitched murmur.

Pulmonary regurgitation is best heard on the right of the sternum, in held inspiration. It has a blowing sound and variable pitch.

The Graham Steell murmur is due to mitral stenosis causing pulmonary hypertension leading to pulmonary hypertension. It is best heard at the left sternal edge.

Systolic murmurs may be divided into ejection systolic, mid-systolic, pansystolic or late systolic.

- Ejection systolic murmurs include: aortic stenosis, pulmonary stenosis, atrial septal defects, hypertrophic cardiomyopathy, Fallot's tetralogy and flow murmurs (from aortic regurgitation or pulmonary regurgitation).
- Pansystolic murmurs include: mitral regurgitation – best heard at the apex to the axilla, flowing in nature; tricuspid regurgitation – best heard at the left sternal edge and low-pitched; ventricular septal defect – heard at the left sternal edge, loud and rough.
- Late systolic murmurs include: hypertrophic obstructive cardial myopathy (note this may also produce an ejection mid-systolic murmur) – this murmur is best heard on standing; mitral valve prolapse – best heard at the apex; coarctation of the aorta – heard at the left sternal edge radiating to the back.

2.34 Large tongue **Answers: B C D**

Amyloid of the AL type causes infiltration and hence enlargement of the tongue.

Acromegaly causes enlargement because of over growth of soft tissues. In Down's syndrome the tongue is said to be fissured and prominent (this may be relative to the size of the mouth rather than a true increase in size). Vitamin B12 deficiency causes a painful red tongue, but it is not enlarged.

2.35 Dementia **Answers: C E**

Dementia is a decline in cognitive function in a setting of clear consciousness. It is usually but not always progressive and with treatment may even be improved.

It is termed pre-senile if it occurs before the age of 60. There is an hereditary pre-disposition to certain dementias and some (e.g. Pick's and Huntington's diseases) have a clear genetic basis.

Environmental agents, such as aluminium, prions and viruses, have also been implicated. Metabolic disorders such as hypothyroidism, vitamin

B12 deficiency, infection (e.g. neurosyphilis), head injury and cerebro-vascular disease (e.g. multiple infarcts) may all cause dementia. It is thus essential to screen for these conditions and commence treatment to prevent further deterioration.

One of the early features of dementia, particularly of the Alzheimer's type, is a reversal of the sleep-wake cycle and patients are seen to wander at night.

The mini mental test score is very helpful, but dementia should not be diagnosed from a single test. A score < 6 should alert the clinician but dementia must be diagnosed on repeated assessments of the patient, interviews with the relatives and after exclusion of the conditions mentioned above.

2.36 Pulmonary tuberculosis **Answers: A E**

Questions on pulmonary TB are extremely common in finals exams.

In the late 1980s the World Health Organization (WHO) declared the rise in incidence of TB to be a global emergency.

Human tuberculosis is caused by infection with *Mycobacterium tuberculosis, M. bovis* or *M. africanum.*

Seventy-five per cent of new cases of TB involve the respiratory system. Pulmonary TB may produce a variety of abnormalities on chest X-ray, including cavitating lesions, hilar enlargement, nodules and consolidation. If the chest X-ray is normal, pulmonary TB is highly unlikely. (TB bronchitis may occur with a normal chest X-ray, but this is extremely rare.)

The diagnosis is made from the history, examination and clinical investigations. Blood cultures are not helpful as the Mycobacterium bacillus cannot be grown from blood. Acid-fast bacilli (AFB) can be obtained from sputum smears and gastric washings and conventionally it takes six weeks for the AFB to grow and drug sensitivities to be obtained. However, newer techniques involving the polymerase chain reaction (PCR) enable the diagnosis to be made more quickly. This is proving to be useful in cases of tuberculosis meningitis where PCR techniques can be applied to CSF samples.

Early morning urine specimens are used to look for renal TB.

Skin testing with the Mantoux or Heaf test may be useful. The Mantoux test involves purified peptide derivative (PPD) preparation being injected intradermally, a result being read 48–72 hours later. The Heaf test involves placing PPD on to the skin and then piercing this area of skin with the six needles of the Heaf gun. The results of the tests are not always conclusive – in overwhelming TB the skin tests may be negative and routine immunisation of many individuals will lead them to have positive results anyway.

However, the Heaf and Mantoux tests are of use in determining which patients should be vaccinated. In general, if the standard concentration of PPD (100 unit/ml) is used then Heaf grades 0 and 1 or a Mantoux response of 0–4 mm indicate a negative response and patients may be offered the BCG immunization in the absence of contraindications. Those with a grade 2 Heaf or a Mantoux reaction of 5–14 mm are considered positive and should not be vaccinated. Non-vaccinated individuals with a Heaf grade 3 or 4 or a Mantoux response >15 mm should be referred for specialist advice and consideration of prophylactic chemotherapy. The BCG vaccination is about 70–75% protective for about 20–30 years.

The treatment for pulmonary TB is frequently reviewed, but at the time of writing involves a six-month regime. The initial phase lasts for two months and consists of daily rifampicin isoniazid, pyrazinamide and ethambutol. The continuation phase lasts for a further four months and consists of daily rifampicin and isoniazid. Ethambutol may be omitted from the initial phase if there is a low risk of resistance to isoniazid.

Isoniazid may cause a peripheral neuropathy and it is customary to prescribe daily pyridoxine to prevent this. Ethambutol used to be a standard treatment, but it causes optic neuritis and is not now routinely used. The main side effect of rifampicin is to alter liver enzymes and if bilirubin becomes elevated rifampicin should be stopped.

2.37 Dark urine **Answers: A C D**

Dark urine may occur due to:

- pigments (e.g. beetroot)
- drugs (e.g. rifampicin)
- haemoglobin and its metabolic products (e.g. bilirubin)
- porphyria (urine darkens on standing)
- intravascular haemolysis (e.g malaria – hence the term ‘black water fever’).

Conjugated bilirubin is water-soluble and appears in the urine but unconjugated urine is colourless. Gilbert's syndrome is an hereditary condition where there is a lack of the conjugating enzyme producing increased unconjugated bilirubin.

Heavy proteinuria can cause the urine to be white and frothy.

2.38 Interferon **Answers: B C D**

The two main forms of interferon used for treatment are alpha and beta interferon. Alpha interferon tends to boost the immune system and is therefore used to aid clearance of chronic viral infections, such as chronic hepatitis B and C. Beta interferon reduces immune-mediated destruction of tissue and has been used in trials in multiple sclerosis. However, its use is controversial; there is a minor reduction in length of stay in hospital for relapses but no reduction in mortality has been demonstrated. The drug is extremely expensive and should only be prescribed by a consultant neurologist.

The side effects of both types of interferon include flu-like symptoms, myalgia and depression. Hepatitis A does not exist in a chronic state.

2.39 Epilepsy **Answers: A B C D E**

It is well known that flashing lights can provoke a seizure. Illness, particularly causing a high fever, may precipitate fits especially in children. Head injury, cerebral infarction and brain tumours are causes of new onset seizures. Anti-convulsant overdose produces cerebellar signs and can increase fit frequency. 'A family argument' is a question that has been reported by many candidates. The answer is true and the explanation is probably that it is due to stress, another well-recognised factor.

2.40 Osteoporosis **Answers: B C D**

Management of osteoporosis includes prevention and treatment.

- Prevention
  Regular exercise throughout life; adequate dietary calcium; HRT when appropriate; moderate alcohol intake and stopping smoking.
- Treatment
  General (i.e. pain relief, physiotherapy)
  Specific (i.e. drugs to stimulate bone formation, e.g. fluoride)
  Drugs to prevent bone resorption (e.g. HRT) – cyclical disodium etridonate with calcium carbonate, calcitonin and calcium.

All patients should receive supplemental calcium and where an additional anti-resorptive agent is indicated the initial choice is between a biphosphonate (e.g. etridonate) and HRT.

2.41 Post-myocardial infarction Answers: A B C D

Although there have been many trials looking at mortality after myocardial infarction, the most important ones to know about are the ISIS (International Study of Infarct Survival) trials.

ISIS I examined the effect of beta-blockade within 12 hours of the onset of chest pain. The result showed a reduction in mortality of 15% at seven days. The mechanism was thought to be prevention of cardiac rupture, reduction of arrhythmia and limitation of infarct size.

ISIS II measured the five-week mortality. Patients were randomised into four groups:

- 1.5 million units of streptokinase – 25% reduction in mortality
- aspirin – 23% reduction in mortality
- streptokinase plus aspirin – 42% reduction in mortality
- placebo

The importance of ISIS II was that the effects of streptokinase and aspirin were additive.

ISIS III looked at different thrombolytic agents. It was found that there was no significant advantage with the newer, more expensive agents and streptokinase was therefore the first-line treatment. However, subsequent studies, including GISSI II and GUSTO, showed the benefit of recombinant tissue plasminogen activator (rTPA).

RTPA should be given to patients who are eligible for thrombolytic therapy who

- have an anterior MI and are under 65 years
- have a known allergy to streptokinase
- a recent (<1 month) proven streptococcal infection
- have had streptokinase >5 days ago and <1 year ago

Note that policies differ between hospitals

ISIS IV examined the effects of ACE inhibition after myocardial infarction. A further 7% reduction in mortality was noted at 5 weeks. Numerous other studies have confirmed the beneficial effect of ACE inhibition. It is now common practice to give ACE inhibitors to patients with clinical evidence of heart failure or impaired LV function (e.g. demonstrated by echocardiography) or who have extensive Q wave infarction.

The role of magnesium is controversial. Some studies supported the use of magnesium, others did not. The question refers to oral magnesium which has not been shown to be of benefit.

2.42 Hypothyroidism **Answers: A B D**

Hypothyroidism is an important endocrine condition with widespread effects on the body.

- Skin (often dry, peripherally cyanosed, cold and swollen; peri-orbital oedema, xanthelasma and associated autoimmune conditions, e.g. vitiligo)
- Cardiovascular system (bradycardia, low volume pulse, pericardial effusion)
- Respiratory system (pleural effusion)
- Central nervous system (speech – this may be slow or hoarse; hearing – nerve deafness which may be bilateral; cognitive function – depression/dementia)
- Peripheral nervous system (proximal myopathy, delayed relaxation of reflex jerks; carpal tunnel syndrome)
- Anaemia (macrocytic – associated with pernicious anaemia; microcytic – iron deficiency, for example, due to menorrhagia)
- Hypercholesterolaemia
- Hypothermia

In the severe form a patient may present in coma and careful thyroxine replacement is necessary.

Hirsutism is not a feature. In fact, loss of hair occurs.

Pre-tibial myxoedema is an unfortunate term because 'myxoedema' is another term for hypothyroidism but in fact this condition occurs in *hyper*thyroidism.

2.43 Mouth ulceration — Answers: A D E

It is worth learning a list of diseases that cause ulceration inside the mouth and diseases that cause genital ulceration as questions are often asked about these.

Causes of oral and/or genital ulceration:

- Behçet's disease
- Reiter's disease
- Crohn's disease
- Strachan's syndrome
- herpes simplex, types 1 and 2
- syphilis
- pemphigus

Ulcerative colitis does not cause oral or genital ulceration, whereas Crohn's disease can cause both. Stress can cause aphthous mouth ulcers but not genital ulcers.

2.44 Colonic carcinoma — Answers: A B C

Familial adenomatous polyposis accounts for 1% of all cases of carcinoma of the colon. (See Paper 1, Question 1.13)

Hereditary non-polyposis colon cancer is an autosomal dominant condition, the gene of which has been localised to chromosome 2. It accounts for 5–15% of cases of carcinoma of the colon. A few adenomatous polyps develop which rapidly transform to cancer.

Ulcerative colitis predisposes to malignancy (after 10 years of colitis, malignant foci in the large bowel are frequent). Crohn's disease is associated with a slight increase in colonic carcinoma, but this is not as common as in ulcerative colitis.

Recent evidence has suggested that constipation allows increased time for carcinogens to lie in contact with the bowel wall, predisposing to malignancy.

Diverticular disease itself does not predispose to malignancy.

2.45 Cerebellopontine angle lesions Answers: A B C D

The key to this question is knowledge of the neuroanatomy. In the cerebellopontine angle are the cerebellar tracts, the Vth, VIIth and VIIIth cranial nerves. From this it can be deduced that tumours in this area may cause facial numbness (damage to V), weakness (damage to VII), deafness (damage to VIII) and ataxia (cerebellar pathway damage).

2.46 Median nerve Answers: A E

The median nerve supplies the muscles of the hand which may be remembered by use of the mnemonic *LOAF:*

Lumbricals I & II
Oponens pollicis
Abductor pollicis
Flexor pollicis brevis

The ulnar nerve supplies the rest of the muscles of the hand, including adduction of the thumb.

Sensation: the lateral 3½ fingers are supplied by the median nerve; the ulnar nerve supplies the medial 1½ fingers.

Tingling in the arm is a common symptom of carpal tunnel syndrome (as is pain in the forearm) but pain in the upper arm is not.

2.47 Care of the elderly Answers: A B C

Altered behaviour/confusion is a common presenting symptom of infection in the elderly; even a urinary tract infection may cause symptoms suggestive of a dementia or even produce a coma. The elderly are more prone to hypothyroidism and sensitivity to the cold encourages them to sit close to fires, producing erythema ab igne.

Part III accommodation is only for people who are continent; incontinent people need to be considered for nursing homes.

A haemoglobin of 10 g/dl is not within the normal range – it is too low. Cardiopulmonary resuscitation should not be on the basis of age.

2.48 Eosinophilia **Answer: A B D E**

The normal eosinophil count is 0.04–0.4 x 10^9/l and may be raised 100- or even 1000-fold in disease states. Causes of eosinophilia include:

- infection – fungi, parasites
- drugs (e.g. sulphonamides, tetracyclines, nitrofurantoin, NSAIDs)
- vasculitis (e.g. Churg-Strauss syndrome, see below) which is defined as asthma, eosinophilia and vasculitis affecting two or more organs apart from the lungs; but any other cause of a vasculitis may cause eosinophilia – e.g. rheumatoid arthritis
- dermatological conditions (e.g. eczema, scabies, pemphigus, pemphigoid)
- malignancy – lymphoproliferative disease, such as Hodgkin's disease; myeloproliferative disease such as hypereosinophilic syndrome.

Churg-Strauss syndrome is defined as asthma, eosinophilia and vasculitis affecting two or more organs apart from the lungs. Any other cause of vasculitis may cause eosinophilia, e.g. rheumatoid arthritis.

2.49 Pleural effusion **Answers: A D**

Oesophageal rupture causes leakage of fluid into the mediastinum and a pleural effusion is common. Liver cirrhosis causes a pleural effusion due to hypo-albuminaemia and the effusion is therefore a transudate. Sarcoid rarely produces a pleural effusion; more commonly it produces reticular nodular shadowing with hilar enlargement and fibrosis.

COAD does not produce a pleural effusion and its presence may be indicative of coexisting heart failure or an underlying malignancy.

Diabetic ketoacidosis does not produce a pleural effusion. In the initial stage the patient is hypovolaemic, but if fluid replacement is excessive then heart failure and pleural effusions may develop.

2.50 Left ventricular failure **Answers: BC D E**

Acute left ventricular failure (LVF) is one of the most important medical emergencies. The patient must be assessed with regard to ABC (i.e. Airway, Breathing and Circulation). If the airway is patent and breathing is adequate, attention needs to be paid to circulation. Intravenous access by use of a large bore cannula must be obtained. The patient needs to be sitting upright breathing 100% oxygen (unless there is a clear history of COAD). Management depends on the state of the patient; for example, if moribund, hypotensive and unable to breathe then ventilation may be appropriate. However, if the patient is well enough, information may be obtained to confirm a history of LVF, i.e. orthopnoea, paroxysmal nocturnal dyspnoea and precipitating factors, such as MI, change of medication or arrhythmia may become apparent.

Examination: the clinical features of LVF include tachycardia with a weak, low volume pulse; a low systolic blood pressure; a displaced apex beat (displaced laterally and inferiorly) and on auscultation a third heart sound may be heard, producing a gallop rhythm. When the heartbeat alternates between good and then poor volume (pulsus alternans) the heart failure is severe and indicates a poor prognosis.

Basic investigations: FBC, U&Es, cardiac enzymes if appropriate, ECG, chest radiograph, temperature and urinalysis.

Drug treatment includes oxygen at the highest concentration tolerated; IV diamorphine (plus anti-emetic). Diamorphine dilates pulmonary veins and therefore reduces the work of the heart and it also relieves the sensation of breathlessness. IV frusemide has a rapid venodilator action in the lungs; its diuretic action takes time to have an effect.

Angiotensin converting enzyme (ACE) inhibitors decrease mortality and morbidity in LVF.

It is worth remembering the pathophysiology of LVF. The heart is a muscular pump. As it fails the heart gets bigger and pumps less efficiently. A back pressure develops and the pulmonary venous pressure rises. As it rises further fluid is squeezed out of the veins into the lung interstitium and can be seen as septal lines (Kerley B lines) and fluid in the horizontal fissure. As the pressure rises further fluid accumulates in the alveoli, giving the typical 'fluffy' shadowing on chest radiography.

The rationale for treatment can therefore be understood. By giving venodilators the pulmonary venous pressure is reduced; diuretics enable the excess fluid to be excreted via the kidneys; ACE inhibitors inhibit angiotensin II mediated vasoconstriction and therefore reduce the workload of the heart; positive inotropes, such as dopamine and dobutamine, increase the contractility of the heart.

2.51 Schizophrenia **Answers: A B C D E**

This question has been reported many times with virtually identical stems each time.

Many drugs of abuse produce a schizophreniform picture. These include amphetamines, opiates, and LSD. There is some suggestion that cannabis may also produce these symptoms.

Temporal lobe epilepsy is a great mimicker; it may produce auditory, olfactory or visual hallucinations.

In pregnancy there is an increased incidence of psychosis, both depressive and schizophrenic.

Hypoglycaemia may produce abnormal bizarre behaviour and is therefore marked 'true'. In this type of question the term 'schizophrenia' can be interpreted loosely as there is no reference to acute or chronic and therefore a broad range of symptoms is covered.

Acute schizophrenia may produce delusions, auditory hallucinations, thought disorders, abnormal affective responses and disordered behaviour.

Schneider's first rank symptoms for diagnosis include:

- thought insertion
- thought broadcasting
- hearing one's thoughts spoken out loud
- auditory hallucinations in the form of a running commentary
- auditory hallucinations in the form of voices discussing the patient in the third person
- feelings of passivity
- primary delusions

Chronic schizophrenia causes slowness, apathy and social withdrawal as well as positive symptoms.

2.52 Hirsutism **Answers: A B C D E**

This is a difficult question. We have used the harder stems from previous papers and put them into one question!

Hirsutism is an increase in body hair. Note that virilism is an increase in body hair in a male distribution. Virilism implies there is hirsutism but the other way round does not apply; a patient may be hirsute but not virilised, whereas a virilised patient is hirsute.

Signs of virilisation include a receding hair line, increased oiliness of the skin, breast atrophy, increased muscle bulk, clitoromegaly, increase in pubic hair and hair on the upper thighs, the lower abdomen, chest, breasts, and the moustache and beard areas. Fine hair on the face, arms and lower legs is not androgen dependent. Virilism is produced by excess androgens which may be adrenal in origin, for example, congenital adrenal hyperplasia, or benign or malignant adrenal tumour. It may be ovarian in origin (for example, tumour, severe polycystic ovarian syndrome) or related to drug administration of androgens.

Hirsutism is caused by:

- all the above
- constitutional (endocrinology is normal, and it may be familial or racial)
- endocrine disorders (e.g. Cushing's syndrome, acromegaly, hyperthyroidism)
- metabolic conditions (e.g. porphyria cutanea tarda)
- drugs (e.g. minoxidil, phenytoin, diazoxide and corticosteroids)
- anorexia nervosa

2.53 Abnormal speech **Answers: A B C D E**

The production of speech is complex and involves pathways from the dominant motor cortex, pathways from the cerebellum for co-ordination of speech, temporal lobe for memory and the actual muscles involved in speech production, for example, larynx, pharynx, tongue and facial muscles. The nerve supply to these muscles may be affected as may the neuromuscular junction. Examples include lesions of the following:

- cerebral cortex (stroke)
- cerebellar (tumour, abscess, infarct, haemorrhage)
- central pathways (e.g. space occupying lesions, demyelination)
- muscles (e.g. motor neurone disease)
- neuromuscular junction (e.g. myasthenia gravis)
- nerve supply (e.g. demyelination)

2.54 Ulcerative colitis **Answers:BCDE**

Both ulcerative colitis and Crohn's disease have extragastrointestinal manifestations.

- Skin – erythema nodosum, pyoderma gangrenosum, vasculitis; note that dermatitis herpetiformis is associated with coeliac disease.
- Eyes – uveitis, episcleritis and conjunctivitis.
- Joints – monoarticular arthritis and sacro-iliitis occur quite frequently in Crohn's disease. Ankylosing spondylitis occurs less commonly, whereas in ulcerative colitis ankylosing spondylitis is more common.
- Abdomen – fatty change of the liver is common in both Crohn's and ulcerative colitis and cirrhosis may occur in both; sclerosing cholangitis is more common in ulcerative colitis.
- Kidney and gall bladder stones occur very frequently in Crohn's disease but not ulcerative colitis.

All the above, apart from liver changes and renal and gall bladder stones are related to disease activity. In general, the presence of colitis in Crohn's disease causes more extra-gastrointestinal complications than if small-bowel lesions alone are present.

2.55 Heart sounds **Answers: A B C**

The second heart sound is caused by the closure of the aortic and pulmonary valves.

The left ventricle finishes emptying before the right heart and therefore the aortic component precedes the pulmonary component. Inspiration increases the venous return to the right heart further delaying right heart emptying and therefore closure of the pulmonary valve. This delay is physiological and is most commonly heard in children or young adults. It becomes abnormal (i.e. widely split in inspiration) when there is a further delay to right heart emptying, for example, RBBB block, pulmonary stenosis.

Left ventricular failure, aortic stenosis and LBBB block delay emptying of the left heart and hence closure of the aortic valve. On inspiration the two sounds are close together but during expiration the right heart empties more quickly and the pulmonary valve closes earlier than the aortic valve giving rise to reverse splitting.

The second heart sound is best heard with the diaphragm placed over the aortic or pulmonary area and the pulmonary component of the second heart sound is really only heard in the pulmonary area. Splitting in the mitral area is not physiological.

Fixed splitting only occurs in an ASD and is therefore pathognomonic. The aortic second sound is louder in systemic hypertension and when a hyperdynamic circulation is present. It is quiet in aortic stenosis because the valve is relatively immobile and in cardiac failure low blood flow also causes a quiet aortic component. Similarly, in pulmonary hypertension the pulmonary component of the second heart sound is loud and it is soft in pulmonary stenosis.

2.56 Tick-borne infection **Answer: D**

Questions about infectious diseases are always extremely difficult and the amount of information to learn seems endless! It is worth knowing about malaria in some detail.
Insect transmission often appears in questions.

- Mosquitoes transmit malaria, dengue, yellow fever, filariasis
- Ticks/fleas carry typhus, Lyme disease, plague
- Flies transmit leishmaniasis, African trypanosomiasis, loiasis, onchocerciasis
- Bugs carry Chagas disease

2.57 Statistics **Answers: C D E**

The mode is the most frequently occurring value in a population. The median is the middle value when the values are ranked in order. The mean is sum of all the observed values divided by the number of values.
In a normal distribution:

$$\text{mean} = \text{mode} = \text{median}$$

The standard deviation (SD) is a measure of the spread of a normally distributed population so that ±1 SD includes 68% of the population, ±2 SD includes 95% and ±3 SD includes 99% of the population.

2.58 Statistics **Answers: B C D**

The standard error of the mean allows calculation of how accurate a sample mean is in estimating the mean of a population.

$$SE = SD/\sqrt{n}$$

where n is the number of values in the sample (not the square). From this a level of confidence can be calculated. The confidence is how close the sample mean is to the population mean. The sample mean ±2 SD is the confidence limit of the mean, i.e. 95% confident that the population mean lies within that range.

A p value of < 0.05 is usually taken to be representative of statistical significance.

The χ^2 test is used to test the difference between two independently derived proportions. It should be performed only on actual numbers of recurrences and not on percentages, proportions or means.

Student's t-test is useful for small samples with a normal distribution. Nonparametric tests are used to analyse data that do not conform to a normal distribution.

A type 1 error suggests that there is statistical significance when there is not and a type 2 error suggests a lack of significance when, in fact, there is significance.

2.59 Photosensitivity **Answers: A B D**

The term 'photosensitivity' implies an abnormal sensitivity of the skin to light (both visible and UV). Implicit in this is an increased risk of skin cancer. The three important conditions producing photosensitivity are:

- SLE
- porphyria (all types except acute intermittent)
- pellagra

By inducing the above conditions, drugs can also produce photosensitivity. For example, lupus may be induced by isoniazid, chlorpromazine, procainamide, hydralazine.

Pellagra may be induced by isoniazid. Oral contraceptives can produce lupus and porphyria. All the above induce photosensitivity indirectly.

Many drugs induce photosensitivity directly, for example, amiodarone, chlorpropamide, sulphonamides, quinine, psoralens. The drug is distributed systemically but interaction with sunlight is necessary so the rash only appears in sun-exposed areas.

2.60 Chorea **Answers: A B C D**

Choreiform movements are sudden involuntary jerky movements. They are due to a lesion of the corpus striatum. The abnormal movements occur more distally compared to hemiballismus which tends to be unilateral and involves the proximal joints and is caused by subthalamic lesions. Athetosis produces a slow writhing movement distally and is due to a lesion of the putamen.

The causes of chorea include:

- hereditary – benign hereditary chorea, Huntington's disease
- acquired endocrine – thyrotoxicosis, pregnancy
- connective tissue – SLE
- metabolic – Wilson's disease
- vascular – vasculitis, stroke
- infectious
  - – bacterial: post-streptococcal infection may produce Sydenham's bacterial chorea, a major criterion for diagnosis of rheumatic fever
  - – viral: viral encephalitis
- drugs – oral contraceptive pill, L-dopa, alcohol
- neoplasia – primary or secondary neoplasia

MULTIPLE CHOICE QUESTION PAPER 3

60 questions: time allowed 2½ hours
Mark your answers with a tick (True) or a cross (False) in the box provided. Leave the box blank for 'Don't know'. Do not look at the answers until you have completed the whole question paper.

3.1 Diabetic patients

❑ A need to inform the DVLA of their condition
❑ B should be given human insulin in preference to porcine insulin
❑ C can now be given insulin orally, avoiding the need for injections
❑ D should stop taking metformin when having an intravenous urogram
❑ E should stop their insulin if they are too ill to eat

3.2 High dose oxygen treatment is advised for a patient with

❑ A acute asthma and a PCO_2 of 3 kPa
❑ B acute asthma and a PCO_2 of 6.5 kPa
❑ C chronic obstructive pulmonary disease
❑ D pneumonia
❑ E pulmonary embolism

3.3 The following are true of lipid lowering drugs:

❑ A the aim of treatment is to raise LDL and lower HDL cholesterol
❑ B they are only effective in secondary prevention of coronary heart disease
❑ C statins are used to treat hypercholesterolaemia
❑ D fibrates are used to treat hypertriglyceridaemia
❑ E fibrates are used to treat mixed hyperlipidaemia

3.4 Primary tumours which commonly metastasise to the lung include

❑ A breast
❑ B brain
❑ C thyroid
❑ D kidney
❑ E prostate

3.5 Infective causes of colitis include

- ❑ A tapeworm infection
- ❑ B salmonella
- ❑ C influenza
- ❑ D *E. coli*
- ❑ E *Clostridium difficile*

3.6 The following are true of audit studies:

- ❑ A they are the same as research
- ❑ B large sample sizes are essential
- ❑ C they are observational
- ❑ D they are susceptible to bias
- ❑ E statistical analysis cannot be performed

3.7 A diabetic patient has an autonomic neuropathy. As a result he may suffer from the following:

- ❑ A nocturnal diarrhoea
- ❑ B postural hypotension
- ❑ C impotence
- ❑ D urine retention
- ❑ E increased sweating

3.8 Causes of Horner's syndrome include

- ❑ A herpes zoster infection
- ❑ B stroke
- ❑ C carotid dissection
- ❑ D lung carcinoma
- ❑ E trauma to the neck

3.9 Investigations which are useful in the diagnosis of myasthenia gravis include

- ❑ A Epsilon test
- ❑ B anticholinesterase antibodies
- ❑ C electromyogram (EMG)
- ❑ D chest X-ray
- ❑ E CT scan of the brain

3.10 Causes of cataract include

- ❑ A increase in age
- ❑ B diabetes mellitus
- ❑ C glaucoma
- ❑ D trauma
- ❑ E prolonged contact lens use

3.11 The following apply to the normal ECG:

- ❑ A it is recorded using 12 electrodes
- ❑ B V4 and V5 record from the interventricular septum
- ❑ C the normal axis is –30 to +90
- ❑ D down-sloping ST depression is a non-specific finding
- ❑ E the PR interval is recorded from the start of the P wave to the R wave peak

3.12 The following are signs of a parietal lobe lesion:

- ❑ A grasp reflex
- ❑ B emotional lability
- ❑ C homonymous quadrantanopia
- ❑ D sensory inattention
- ❑ E difficulty calculating numbers

3.13 Pulmonary fibrosis is a recognised sequel to

- ❑ A sarcoidosis
- ❑ B rheumatoid arthritis
- ❑ C radiotherapy
- ❑ D asbestosis
- ❑ E emphysema

3.14 Features of multiple myeloma include

- ❑ A fractures
- ❑ B hypercalcaemia
- ❑ C renal failure
- ❑ D raised alkaline phosphatase
- ❑ E hypogammaglobulinaemia

3.15 Raynaud's phenomenon is a recognised feature of

- ❑ A cryoglobulinaemia
- ❑ B scleroderma
- ❑ C diabetes mellitus
- ❑ D cervical rib
- ❑ E Buerger's disease

3.16 Features of Zollinger-Ellison syndrome include

- ❑ A metabolic acidosis
- ❑ B multiple peptic ulcers
- ❑ C high gastric acid levels
- ❑ D low serum gastrin
- ❑ E malignant potential

3.17 Neuropathic joints may occur in

- ❑ A tuberculosis
- ❑ B yaws
- ❑ C leprosy
- ❑ D syringomyelia
- ❑ E tabes dorsalis

3.18 Recurrent renal stones may be due to

- ❑ A hypoparathyroidism
- ❑ B high protein intake
- ❑ C cystinuria
- ❑ D Crohn's disease
- ❑ E hot climate

3.19 Positive test for rheumatoid factor occurs in

- ❑ A Reiter's syndrome
- ❑ B chronic gout
- ❑ C Still's disease
- ❑ D Sjögren's syndrome
- ❑ E SLE

3.20 Recognised causes of pyrexia include

- ❑ A neuroleptic drugs
- ❑ B Hodgkin's lymphoma
- ❑ C basal cell carcinoma
- ❑ D connective tissue disorders
- ❑ E hypothyroidism

3.21 The following commonly occur in heart failure:

- ❑ A a boot-shaped heart on chest radiograph
- ❑ B fine basal crepitations in the lung
- ❑ C pleural effusion
- ❑ D large pulmonary vessels
- ❑ E haemoptysis

3.22 The following imply that a bronchial carcinoma has metastasised:

- ❑ A hyponatraemia
- ❑ B peripheral neuropathy
- ❑ C ptosis
- ❑ D ataxia
- ❑ E small-muscle wasting

3.23 Lower respiratory tract infections are more common in

- ❑ A Crohn's disease
- ❑ B Down's syndrome
- ❑ C emphysema
- ❑ D motor neurone disease
- ❑ E Duchenne muscular dystrophy

3.24 Thrombocytopenia occurs in

- ❑ A chronic lymphocytic leukaemia
- ❑ B myelofibrosis
- ❑ C SLE
- ❑ D prolonged aspirin therapy
- ❑ E acromegaly

3.25 Erectile dysfunction may result from

- ❑ A a transurethral resection of the prostate
- ❑ B cimetidine therapy
- ❑ C depression
- ❑ D diabetes mellitus
- ❑ E chronic alcohol consumption

3.26 Chronic bronchitis may cause

- ❑ A a raised arterial PCO_2
- ❑ B a decreased arterial PO_2
- ❑ C a raised haematocrit
- ❑ D a raised hemidiaphragm on chest X-ray
- ❑ E a raised pulmonary arterial pressure

3.27 The following cause a loud first heart sound:

- ❑ A mitral stenosis
- ❑ B emphysema
- ❑ C anaemia
- ❑ D thin patient
- ❑ E heart failure

3.28 The following are causes of atrial fibrillation:

- ❑ A chest infection
- ❑ B alcoholism
- ❑ C myocardial infarction
- ❑ D mitral valve regurgitation
- ❑ E myxoedema

3.29 The following may provide a clue to the aetiology of hypertension in a patient:

- ❑ A systolic murmur near the midline of the back
- ❑ B episodic muscular weakness
- ❑ C AV nipping in the retinal vessels
- ❑ D neurofibromas
- ❑ E tall R waves in V6

3.30 Jaundice producing dark urine occurs in

- ❑ A Gilbert's syndrome
- ❑ B thalassaemia
- ❑ C carcinoma of the head of the pancreas
- ❑ D nitrazepam-induced jaundice
- ❑ E breast milk jaundice

3.31 In a cardiac arrest

- ❑ A 28% oxygen should be administered via a face mask until an anaesthetist arrives
- ❑ B the ratio of cardiac compressions to ventilations is 15:2
- ❑ C 1 mg of adrenaline should be administered intravenously every 3 mins irrespective of the cardiac rhythm
- ❑ D if the underlying rhythm is VF, 3 minutes of CPR should be performed between sequences of 3 shocks
- ❑ E atropine should be given in asystole

3.32 Referral to an ophthalmologist is essential for all diabetic patients with

- ❑ A one microaneurysm
- ❑ B one cotton wool spot
- ❑ C one blot haemorrhage
- ❑ D one hard exudate
- ❑ E maculopathy

3.33 Regarding ventricular fibrillation

- ❑ A DC shock must not be attempted more than six times because of damage to the myocardium
- ❑ B a central pulse may be present
- ❑ C it may occur as a result of myocardial infarction
- ❑ D the prognosis is better than for asystole
- ❑ E treatment should be abandoned after 5 minutes of ventricular fibrillation as defibrillation after this time is unlikely to be successful

3.34 The following predispose to UTI:

- ❑ A renal calculi
- ❑ B catheterisation
- ❑ C post-general anaesthetic
- ❑ D double ureter
- ❑ E being female

3.35 Causes of a round face include

- ❑ A Cushing's syndrome
- ❑ B acromegaly
- ❑ C obesity
- ❑ D muscular dystrophy
- ❑ E nephrotic syndrome

3.36 In nephrotic syndrome

- ❑ A there is an increased risk of infection
- ❑ B hypogammaglobulinaemia is diagnostic
- ❑ C venous thrombosis is common
- ❑ D children have a better outcome
- ❑ E renal failure will eventually occur

3.37 After pituitary ablation in a male the following must always be replaced:

- ❑ A hydrocortisone
- ❑ B glucagon
- ❑ C thyroxine
- ❑ D testosterone
- ❑ E growth hormone

3.38 Patients with hypertension have an increased risk of

- ❑ A haemorrhagic stroke
- ❑ B embolic stroke
- ❑ C myocardial infarction
- ❑ D left ventricular failure
- ❑ E aortic stenosis

3.39 The following occur in nutritional rickets:

- ❑ A raised serum alkaline phosphatase
- ❑ B lowered plasma calcium
- ❑ C raised serum phosphate
- ❑ D raised serum PTH
- ❑ E enlargement of the costochondral junction

3.40 Swelling of the arm may be caused by

- ❑ A SVC obstruction
- ❑ B breast surgery
- ❑ C radiotherapy
- ❑ D ipsilateral stroke
- ❑ E aortic dissection

3.41 Asbestos exposure may cause

- ❑ A left ventricular failure
- ❑ B bronchial carcinoma
- ❑ C lung fibrosis
- ❑ D mesothelioma
- ❑ E pleural and peritoneal plaques

3.42 Bone metastases are commonly produced by the following cancers:

- ❑ A prostate
- ❑ B thyroid
- ❑ C breast
- ❑ D ovary
- ❑ E brain

3.43 Weight loss of over 6.5 kg in 2 months may be due to

- ❑ A depression
- ❑ B anxiety
- ❑ C bronchial adenoma
- ❑ D hyperthyroidism
- ❑ E diabetes mellitus

3.44 Causes of clinically significant weight gain include

❑ A nephrotic syndrome
❑ B bronchial carcinoma
❑ C pelvic malignancy
❑ D congestive cardiac failure
❑ E diabetes insipidus

3.45 Causes of absent ankle jerk reflexes include

❑ A old age
❑ B diabetes mellitus
❑ C syphilis
❑ D motor neurone disease
❑ E Parkinson's disease

3.46 A bowed tibia may be due to

❑ A Paget's disease
❑ B osteoporosis
❑ C rickets
❑ D syphilis
❑ E rheumatoid arthritis

3.47 Polyuria and polydipsia may be due to

❑ A hypokalaemia
❑ B hypocalcaemia
❑ C diabetes mellitus
❑ D acute renal failure
❑ E diabetes insipidus

3.48 A generalised change in skin colour occurs with

❑ A pernicious anaemia
❑ B haemochromatosis
❑ C hypercarotinaemia
❑ D carbon monoxide poisoning
❑ E lead poisoning

3.49 Vomiting may result from

- ❑ A hip surgery
- ❑ B low serum potassium
- ❑ C opiate use
- ❑ D caecal carcinoma
- ❑ E Menière's disease

3.50 Features suggestive of a diagnosis of irritable bowel syndrome include

- ❑ A weight loss
- ❑ B change in bowel habit
- ❑ C small amounts of blood from the rectum
- ❑ D improvement on a gluten-free diet
- ❑ E dysphagia

3.51 The following diseases are paired with appropriate investigations:

❑	A	sarcoid	thallium scan
❑	B	myocardial ischaemia	gallium scan
❑	C	left ventricular function	MUGA scan
❑	D	lung metastases	MRI
❑	E	caecal carcinoma	ultrasound

3.52 Scalp hair may decrease with

- ❑ A hypothyroidism
- ❑ B hypopituitarism
- ❑ C minoxidil tablets
- ❑ D stress
- ❑ E cisplatin

3.53 Which of the following are good screening tests:

- ❑ A faecal occult bloods for a GI malignancy
- ❑ B genetic tests for breast cancer
- ❑ C random cortisol for Cushing's syndrome
- ❑ D resting ECG for asymptomatic coronary artery disease
- ❑ E CA125 for ovarian carcinoma

3.54 The following statements are true concerning the prevalence of a disease:

- ❑ A it is determined from a longitudinal study
- ❑ B it is determined from cross-sectional studies
- ❑ C it depends on the duration of the illness
- ❑ D it is equal to the mortality rate when the case fatality ratio is high
- ❑ E for asthma it is 25%

3.55 A low serum iron and low total iron binding capacity may occur with

- ❑ A rheumatoid arthritis
- ❑ B anaemia of chronic disease
- ❑ C hereditary spherocytosis
- ❑ D iron deficiency
- ❑ E pernicious anaemia

3.56 A raised faecal fat may occur with

- ❑ A ulcerative colitis
- ❑ B subtotal villous atrophy
- ❑ C gallstones
- ❑ D chronic pancreatitis
- ❑ E gastrin-secreting tumour

3.57 Pleural effusion occurs with

- ❑ A oesophagitis
- ❑ B tuberculosis
- ❑ C rheumatoid arthritis
- ❑ D aortic valve replacement
- ❑ E rheumatic fever

3.58 Generalised lymphadenopathy may be caused by

- ❑ A glandular fever
- ❑ B mumps
- ❑ C syphilis
- ❑ D multiple myeloma
- ❑ E HIV infection

3.59 The following are examined in order to certify death:

- ❑ A jugular venous pressure
- ❑ B heart sounds
- ❑ C radial pulse
- ❑ D response to external stimuli
- ❑ E breath sounds

3.60 Angina pectoris may be precipitated by

- ❑ A anaemia
- ❑ B a large meal
- ❑ C watching a violent television programme
- ❑ D thyroxine
- ❑ E acute myocardial infarction

END

Go over your answers until your time is up.
Correct answers and teaching notes are overleaf.

MULTIPLE CHOICE QUESTION PAPER 3 – ANSWERS

The correct answer options for each question are given below.

3.1	A D	3.31	B C E
3.2	A B D E	3.32	B E
3.3	C D E	3.33	C D
3.4	A C D	3.34	A B C D E
3.5	B D E	3.35	A C E
3.6	C D	3.36	A C D
3.7	A B C D	3.37	A C D
3.8	B C D E	3.38	A B C D
3.9	C D	3.39	A B D
3.10	A B C D	3.40	A B C D
3.11	C	3.41	B C D E
3.12	C D E	3.42	A B C
3.13	A B C D	3.43	A D E
3.14	A B C D	3.44	A C D
3.15	A B D	3.45	A B C D
3.16	A B C E	3.46	A C D
3.17	B C D E	3.47	A C E
3.18	B C D E	3.48	A C D
3.19	D E	3.49	A C D E
3.20	A B D	3.50	All false
3.21	B C D E	3.51	C
3.22	All false	3.52	A B D E
3.23	B C D E	3.53	E
3.24	A B C	3.54	B C
3.25	A C D E	3.55	A B
3.26	A B C E	3.56	B D E
3.27	A C D	3.57	B C D
3.28	A B C D	3.58	A C E
3.29	A B D	3.59	B D E
3.30	C D	3.60	A B C D

MCQ PAPER 3 – ANSWERS AND TEACHING NOTES

3.1 Diabetic patients **Answers: A D**

Drivers treated with insulin or oral diabetic drugs are required to notify the DVLA of their condition. Drivers of heavy goods vehicles or public service vehicles whose diabetes is controlled by diet alone must also notify the DVLA.

Insulin may be extracted from pork or beef pancreas but beef insulins are rarely used. Human sequence insulin may be produced by enzymatic modification of porcine insulin or synthetically by DNA technology. All insulin preparations are immunogenic in humans but this rarely causes a problem in clinical practice. It was thought that human insulin would have many advantages over porcine insulin but this has not been established in clinical trials. In fact, some patients have found that switching to human insulin after having had porcine insulin has caused a reduction in the warning symptoms of hypoglycaemia and these patients have been put back on porcine insulin.

Insulin is inactivated by gastro-intestinal enzymes and cannot be given orally. It must be given by injection.

During illness stress hormones such as cortisol cause blood glucose levels to rise. During an illness a diabetic patient is particularly at risk of hyperglycaemia even if they are not eating, and insulin is absolutely necessary. In fact higher doses may be needed.

Diabetic patients taking metformin are at increased risk of lactic acidosis when radiological intravenous contrast agents are given. Most radiology departments recommend that metformin is stopped for 48 hours after performing a procedure such as intravenous urogram and renal function should be checked before restarting the metformin.

3.2 High dose oxygen **Answers: A B D E**

In conditions where hypoventilation is likely, such as chronic obstructive pulmonary disease, high dose oxygen must not be given. Hypoventilation produces a rise in CO_2 and a fall in PO_2; in time the respiratory centres within the brain are reset to tolerate a chronically high PCO_2 and so these patients then rely on their low PO_2 to produce a hypoxic drive for ventilation; if high concentration oxygen is given this drive is abolished and the patient may stop breathing altogether.

High dose oxygen (i.e. up to a concentration of 60%) is appropriate when conditions produce hyperventilation such as an acute asthmatic attack, pneumonia, pulmonary embolism and fibrosing alveolitis. In these conditions a low partial pressure of oxygen is associated with a normal or low PCO_2.

An important exception is a life threatening attack of asthma. The patient may become so exhausted that hypoventilation results, causing a decrease in arterial oxygen tension and a rise in PCO_2. In this case a high concentration of oxygen is required despite the hypoventilation (this is an acute situation and the patient does not normally rely on a hypoxic drive) and positive pressure ventilation should be urgently considered.

3.3 Lipid lowering drugs **Answers: C D E**

Lowering the concentration of low-density lipoprotein (LDL) cholesterol and raising high density (HDL) cholesterol reduces the progression of coronary atherosclerosis and may even induce regression.

There is evidence that if LDL cholesterol can be lowered by 25% – 35%, primary and secondary prevention of coronary heart disease is achieved. Treatment with statins has been shown to reduce myocardial infarction, coronary deaths and overall mortality.

Statins are drugs of first choice for treating hypercholesterolaemia and fibrates for treating hyper-triglyceridaemia. Statins and fibrates can also be used either together or alone to treat mixed hyperlipidaemia.

3.4 Primary tumours **Answers: A C D**

There are four important tumours which commonly metastasise to the lungs. These are carcinoma of the breast, carcinoma of the bronchus, thyroid cancer and renal cancer. Note that this is the same list as metastasise to the bone, with the exception of prostate cancer which does not commonly metastasise to the lung but commonly metastasises to bone.

3.5 Colitis **Answers: B D E**

Infective causes of colitis include Amoebiosis, Shigella, Salmonella, Yersinia, Campylobacter, E. coli 0157 E. and *Clostridium difficile* (pseudo-membranous colitis).

In immuno-compromised hosts other infections such as cytomegalovirus and herpes should also be considered.

Tapeworm infection causes anaemia and weight loss. Influenza is a respiratory tract infection and does not affect the colon.

Other causes of colitis include inflammatory bowel disease, radiation, ischaemic colitis and drugs such as gold.

3.6 Audit studies **Answers: C D**

All doctors are now expected to perform audit studies. Audit will also form part of an annual appraisal of each senior hospital doctor as part of clinical governance which is the legal responsibility of all trusts. Appraisal will also be necessary for revalidation – that is the process where each doctor will submit a profile of their performance to the GMC in order to stay on the Medical Register. This revalidation process will be done every 5 years.

Audit is therefore extremely important to each doctor (and medical students who are also being asked to perform audit studies).

Audit involves the following:

- a standard should be selected e.g. all discharge summaries should be done within two days of the patient's discharge from hospital
- assess the local practice e.g. patients discharged last week
- compare with the target
- implement change
- re-audit to assess whether improvement has occurred

Audit is not research and there are many important differences. Research is more precise, involves larger sample sizes and a longer timescale and has strictly defined methodology. Research compares different things whereas audit is comparing the same activities. Research is experimental whereas audit is observational, making it very susceptible to bias. A good audit study should have a standard error and confidence intervals.

3.7 Autonomic neuropathy **Answers: A B C D**

One of the complications of diabetes mellitus is an autonomic neuropathy. The features of this include postural hypotension, loss of sinus arrhythmia, (pulse does not slow in response to the Valsalva manoeuvre), loss of sweating, impotence, nocturnal diarrhoea, urine retention and incontinence.

3.8 Horner's syndrome **Answers: B C D E**

Horner's syndrome consists of ptosis and a constricted pupil (meiosis). Enophthalmos (the eye appears sunken) and anhidrosis (absence of sweating) may also be present. The sympathetic nervous system has a complicated pathway, and damage at various sites will result in a Horner's syndrome. For example, carcinoma of the lung apex may damage the T1 sympathetic ganglion. A thyroid malignancy or trauma to the neck will damage the sympathetic fibres here. A carotid arterial lesion such as a carotid aneurysm or dissection or peri-carotid tumour would have a similar effect. Brain stem lesions such as a stroke, syringobulbia and tumour can also result in a Horner's syndrome. Syringomyelia is a rare lesion affecting the upper cervical chord and may cause a bilateral Horner's syndrome.

Herpes zoster infection of the geniculate ganglion results in a facial nerve palsy and not Horner's syndrome.

3.9 Myasthenia gravis **Answers: C D**

Tests for myasthenia gravis include:

- Tensilon test – edrophonium is given intravenously and if muscle strength improves dramatically myasthenia gravis is likely
- Acetylcholine receptor antibodies – these occur in up to 90% of cases and false positive results are rare. Anti-striated muscle antibody is detectable in 90% of patients with thymoma but is not a specific test
- Electromyogram – in myasthenia gravis repetitive stimulation at low frequency causes a progressive reduction in muscle action potential amplitudes if that particular muscle is affected
- Investigation for the presence of a thymoma include a chest X-ray and thoracic CT scan

3.10 Cataract **Answers: A B C D**

The likelihood of developing a cataract increases with age. Causes include diabetes mellitus and Cushing's syndrome. Steroids will also increase the risk of cataract formation. Ocular disease such as glaucoma, irradiation and trauma to the eye are also causes. Hereditary or congenital cataracts occur in conditions such as dystrophia myotonica.

3.11 Electrocardiogram **Answer: C**

Although it is known as the 12-lead ECG this refers to 12 vectors. Only 10 electrodes are actually used to obtain these so-called 12 leads. V1 selects activity in the right ventricle, V3–V4 in the interventricular septum and V5–V6 in the left ventricle. 2, 3 and AVF record from the inferior surface and 1, AVL and V6 face the lateral wall of the left ventricle. The normal axis is –30 to +90. Less than -30 would indicate left axis deviation and greater than +90 indicates right axis deviation.

Up-sloping depression is a non-specific finding; down-sloping or planar ST depression >1 mm indicates myocardial ischaemia.

The PR interval is recorded from the start of the P wave to the start of the QRS complex. The ST segment is the period between the end of the QRS complex and the start of the T wave.

3.12 Parietal lobe lesion **Answers: C D E**

Primitive reflexes, such as the grasp reflex and rooting reflex, are signs of a frontal lobe lesion. Other signs of frontal lobe lesion include emotional lability, intellectual impairment, personality change, urinary incontinence and mono- or hemiparesis. Damage to the left frontal region produces Broca's aphasia.

Parietal lobe lesions produce a variety of signs. Damage to either parietal lobe will produce contralateral sensory loss or neglect (another term is sensory hemi-inattention). Constructional apraxia, agraphaesthesia, a failure to recognise surroundings, limb apraxia and homonymous field defect are also signs. The homonymous defect affecting the parietal lobe alone will produce a homonymous quadrantanopia affecting the lower quadrant compared with an upper field defect which occurs with a temporal lobe lesion.

Specific damage to the right parietal region causes a dressing apraxia, and a failure to recognise faces, as well as the above. Damage to the left parietal region can produce Gerstmann's syndrome, consisting of dyscalculia, dysgraphia and left to right disorientation. Although it is not scientific and should not be quoted in an exam, it is helpful to think of the parietal lobes as being responsible for position in space and in addition to this the right lobe is also concerned with the artistic sociable side, whereas the left is the more studious and mathematical side.

3.13 Pulmonary fibrosis **Answers: A B C D**

There are many causes of pulmonary fibrosis and it is helpful to think of causes of upper zone fibrosis separately from mid/lower zone fibrosis.

Causes of upper zone fibrosis can be remembered by the mnemonic *BREAST:*

Berylliosis
Radiation
Extrinsic allergic alveolitis
Ankylosing spondylitis
Sarcoid
TB

Of all of these, the most important at undergraduate level are TB and sarcoidosis.

Lower zone shadowing is caused by the connective tissue diseases, for example, lupus, rheumatoid arthritis, scleroderma; drugs such as cytotoxics, amiodarone, nitrofurantoin; the occupational lung diseases, for example, silicosis, asbestosis.

Pulmonary fibrosis is not caused by emphysema, chronic bronchitis or asthma.

3.14 Multiple myeloma **Answers: A B C D**

Multiple myeloma is due to a monoclonal neoplastic proliferation of plasma cells. These produce abnormal paraprotein which causes hyper-gammaglobulinaemia (because the total immunoglobulin is measured). However, the abnormal globulin suppresses the useful globulin resulting in immune paresis and hence susceptibility to infection. The paraprotein is usually IgG. It may spill over into the urine causing Bence-Jones proteinuria. The bone marrow is unable to function properly and anaemia, neutropenia and thrombocytopenia occur commonly. The malignant plasma cells in the marrow also cause bone destruction resulting in pathological fractures, hypercalcaemia and raised alkaline phosphatase.

The diagnosis is made by:

- FBC – looking for the above
- serum electrophoresis – this will show the abnormal paraprotein
- ESR – this is considerably raised
- U&Es, creatinine – renal failure is caused by paraprotein deposition in the renal tubules

- alkaline phosphatase and calcium – because of bone damage
- urine – Bence-Jones protein
- skeletal survey – multiple lytic lesions may be apparent, particularly in the skull, pelvis, and long bones
- bone marrow biopsy – >10% of the plasma cells in the marrow are malignant.

Serum electrophoresis, skeletal survey and bone marrow biopsy are the most significant investigations for diagnosis.

3.15 Raynaud's phenomenon **Answers: A B D**

Raynaud's phenomenon consists of spasm of the arteries supplying the fingers and toes causing a characteristic colour change, the order of which can be remembered by the mnemonic *WBC* (white blood cell):

White
Blue
Crimson (red)

Raynaud's phenomenon is a common disease affecting 5% of the population, occurring predominantly in young women. It is usually bilateral and the fingers are affected more commonly than the toes. It is precipitated by cold and relieved by warmth. Causes include connective tissue disorders, particularly systemic sclerosis, cryoglobulinaemia, side effect of beta-blocking drugs, presence of a cervical rib and working with vibrating tools. If there is no underlying cause, the term Raynaud's **disease** is used rather than Raynaud's phenomenon.

Treatment:

- treatment of the underlying disease
- stop smoking
- precipitating drugs should be avoided and the hands and feet should be kept warm; electrically heated gloves and socks may help; nifedipine, a vasodilator, may also be used.

Diabetes mellitus affects both the large and small blood vessels, but does not specifically produce Raynaud's phenomenon.

Buerger's disease is a condition found in young men who smoke, causing inflammation of the small vessels of the lower limbs. It may be severe enough to require amputation.

3.16 Zollinger-Ellison syndrome Answers: A B C E

Zollinger-Ellison syndrome is due to a gastrin-secreting tumour that usually arises from G cells in the pancreas. The secretion of gastrin is autonomous and a raised serum gastrin occurs. This in turn produces high levels of acid with the following consequences:

- multiple duodenal ulceration
- metabolic acidosis
- diarrhoea (stimulated by the low pH in the upper intestine)

Patients may present with diarrhoea, or abdominal pain, ulceration and the complications of ulceration, such as haemorrhage and perforation. Omeprazole is the mainstay of treatment although surgery to remove the primary tumour may be performed. The tumour is malignant but slow growing. The syndrome may be part of the wider MEN syndrome involving pituitary tumours, parathyroid adenomas and pancreatic tumours.

3.17 Neuropathic joints Answers: B C D E

A neuropathic or Charcot's joint is a grossly disorganised, but painless joint. It is caused by loss of sensory nerve supply of a joint and hence loss of protective pain sensation. The joint is characteristically swollen with abnormal but painless movement. Causes include tabes dorsalis, syringomyelia, diabetes mellitus, subacute combined degeneration, leprosy and yaws. Tuberculosis may cause painful destruction of a joint.

3.18 Renal stones Answers: B C D E

Important causes of urinary tract stone formation include dehydration; for example, living in a hot climate, multiple myeloma or prolonged illness. Metabolic disturbances include hypercalcaemia (e.g. hyperparathyroidism, sarcoidosis, malignancy); increased oxalate, such as in Crohn's disease; increased uric acid levels; for example, a high protein diet may cause uric acid deposition in the joints causing gout or in the kidney causing stones; cystinuria – produces cystine stones.

Note that stones can cause infection and vice versa.

Stones may also be caused by renal disease, such as renal tubular acidosis.

3.19 Rheumatoid factor **Answers: D E**

A positive test for rheumatoid factor may occur in rheumatoid arthritis, Sjögren's syndrome, SLE, systemic sclerosis, mixed connective tissue disease and polymyositis.

3.20 Pyrexia **Answers: A B D**

There are many causes of pyrexia and although it is tempting to think of infection as the cause, the wide differential must be remembered. Causes include:

- infection
- inflammation (e.g. inflammatory bowel disease)
- malignancy – lymphomas, leukaemias and carcinoma of the liver, pancreas and kidney particularly produce fever, but any disseminated malignancy may also do so. Localised skin tumour, such as basal cell carcinoma, is unlikely to cause a fever unless there is coexisting infection
- connective tissue disorders (e.g. SLE, rheumatoid arthritis)
- vasculitis (e.g. polyarteritis nodosa, sarcoidosis)
- drugs – neuroleptic drugs, such as chlorpromazine, may cause neuroleptic malignant syndrome which causes a very high fever; allergic drug reactions will also produce a fever
- aspirin overdose can produce a hyperpyrexia
- endocrine (e.g. thyroid storm – hypothyroidism produces hypothermia)
- hypothalamic lesions – the central control of temperature is here.

3.21 Heart failure **Answers: B C D E**

(See also the answer to Paper 2, Question 2.50.)

As the left ventricle fails, blood is not pumped out of the heart effectively, causing an increase in pressure in the left ventricle. This is transmitted back to the left atrium and then the pulmonary veins.

On a chest X-ray this can be seen, at first, as an increase in heart size. An increase in both the size and number of upper lobe blood vessels then occurs and as the pressure increases further, fluid leaks into the lung interstitium where it appears as fluid in the horizontal fissure, septal lines, etc, or as a pleural effusion. Further pressure rises causes fluid in the alveoli, i.e. alveolar oedema.

The raised pulmonary venous pressure may cause more vessels to rupture producing haemoptysis (usually small). As the left ventricle fails it enlarges and on chest X-ray the cardiothoracic ratio increases. However, nothing further can be said about the shape of the heart; a boot-shaped heart occurs in Fallot's tetralogy.

3.22 Bronchial carcinoma **Answer: All false**

This question illustrates the wide variety of effects that a bronchial malignancy may have.

- Compression, effusion or obstruction
  Nerve compression
    cervical sympathetic nerve – producing Horner's syndrome
    recurrent laryngeal nerve damage – producing voice hoarseness
    phrenic nerve damage – producing an elevated hemidiaphragm
    T1 nerve damage – leading to small-muscle wasting
  Vessel compression
    artery or vein (e.g. superior vena caval obstruction)
  Pleural effusion
    empyema
  Airway obstruction
    stridor
    collapse
    distal infection
    air trapping
- Metastases
  Discrete lung metastases or hilar node metastases
    brain, liver, adrenal glands, bone
- Non-metastatic effects
  Hormone secretion – especially oat cell tumours –
    ACTH (Cushing's syndrome), PT (hypercalcaemia),
    ADH (hyponatraemia)
  Skin changes (e.g. erythema gyratum repens)
  Hypotrophic pulmonary osteoarthropathy and clubbing
  Neuropathy, myopathy, cachexia, weight loss
  Ataxia – this may be a paraneoplastic phenomenon and therefore does not imply cerebellar metastases, although these should also be considered.

3.23 Lower respiratory tract infections — Answers: B C D E

An increase in incidence of lower respiratory tract infections is seen in:

- primary lung disease (e.g. bronchiectasis, bronchitis, emphysema)
- cardiac disease (e.g. septal defects, pulmonary hypertension; Down's syndrome patients have a higher incidence of these defects)
- neuromuscular disorders, e.g. motor neurone disease – these patients are at risk of aspiration due to bulbar damage and also have difficulty ventilating their lungs due to thoracic wall muscle involvement and diaphragmatic paresis. In myasthenia gravis, fatigue may prevent adequate coughing
- mechanical restriction to adequate lung ventilation, for example, Duchenne muscular dystrophy, polio, ankylosing spondylitis and conditions producing a kyphoscoliosis.

3.24 Thrombocytopenia — Answers: A B C

Thrombocytopenia is defined as a platelet count of less than 150×10^9/l. Causes include:

- Decreased production
  Bone marrow failure due to drugs or malignancy, such as leukaemia
  Megaloblastic anaemia (e.g. vitamin B12 or folate deficiency) results in decreased marrow function
  Uraemia has a deleterious effect on marrow, producing thrombocytopenia
  Alcohol appears to have numerous effects on bone marrow, including direct suppression of function by a toxic effect
  B12/folate deficiency leads to megaloblastic anaemia
  Cirrhosis produces portal hypertension and splenomegaly, the latter causing thrombocytopenia
  Viral infections (e.g. measles, CMV) can inhibit platelet production
- Decreased survival
  For example, immunological autoantibodies are formed against the platelets resulting in their premature destruction; this occurs in conditions such as SLE, chronic lymphatic leukaemia and ITP (idiopathic thrombocytopenic purpura). Some mechanisms of drug-mediated thrombocytopenia are thought to be autoimmune (e.g. heparin, sulphonamides, quinine).
- Increased consumption
  DIC (disseminated intravascular coagulation); sequestration in the spleen (e.g. liver cirrhosis and portal hypertension); massive haemorrhage.

Note that aspirin causes platelet dysfunction but not thrombocytopenia; other drugs with effects on platelets similar to aspirin include indomethacin and streptokinase.

Note that platelet dysfunction may occur despite a normal or even high platelet count. For example, in renal failure and hepatic failure the platelet count may be reduced as mentioned above, or it may be normal with a qualitative defect. In myeloproliferative disorders thrombocythaemia may occur, i.e. an increase in platelets occurs, but the platelet function is abnormal.

3.25 Erectile dysfunction **Answers: A C D E**

Erectile dysfunction (impotence) may result from damage to the nerve or vessels supplying the penis. Nerve damage may follow transurethral resection of the prostate (TURP) and patients must be warned of this. Drug therapy, for example, with beta-blockers, alpha-blockers and thiazide diuretics, may also cause this.

In diabetes mellitus, autonomic nerve damage may occur; the parasympathetic nervous system is responsible for erection and sympathetic nerve for ejaculation. Chronic alcohol consumption will also cause erectile impotence. The higher centres also have an important role and anxiety or depression may produce impotence.

Cystic fibrosis causes infertility in males but not impotence.

3.26 Chronic bronchitis **Answers: A B C E**

Patients with chronic bronchitis are often hypoxic. Mucus plugging in the airways and damage to their walls, together with loss of elastic recoil (as in emphysema), producing early closure of the airways during expiration all contribute to this hypoxia. Unless the patient can hyperventilate, the PCO_2 will also rise, producing a respiratory acidosis. The kidneys retain bicarbonate to normalise the pH so in the chronic state a patient with chronic bronchitis and PCO_2 retention has a raised PCO_2, raised plasma bicarbonate and normal pH (i.e. a compensated respiratory acidosis).

Hypoxia has an important effect; it acts as a stimulus for erythropoietin production by the kidney and polycythaemia produces a rise in haematocrit. The latter can be such a problem as to warrant regular venesection in order to prevent complications such as stroke.

Hypoxia in an area of lung causes vasoconstriction of the blood vessels in that area. This is a protective response in that it diverts blood flow from areas of poor ventilation to those that are better ventilated. However, in the long term, chronic vasoconstriction produces changes in the vessel walls causing a rise in pulmonary arterial pressure. This can eventually lead to cor pulmonale (i.e. right heart failure secondary to lung disease).

A raised hemidiaphragm on a chest X-ray should not be attributed to chronic bronchitis alone. A coexisting lung lesion should be suspected.

3.27 Heart sounds **Answers: A C D**

The first heart sound is loud in:

- thin patients
- hyperdynamic circulation (e.g. thyrotoxicosis or severe anaemia)
- mitral stenosis
- short PR interval

The heart sound is soft in obese patients; in pericardial effusion or tamponade; in emphysema; in cardiac failure when the PR interval is long and in mitral valve regurgitation (valve closure produces the first heart sound and therefore if the valve does not close properly the heart sound is quiet).

3.28 Atrial fibrillation **Answers: A B C D**

There are many causes of atrial fibrillation; the most important ones are ischaemic heart disease, rheumatic heart disease and thyrotoxicosis. The important causes can be considered under the following headings:

- Cardiac causes
  valve disease (e.g. mitral valve disease – whatever the cause)
  conduction abnormality (e.g. Wolf- Parkinson-White syndrome)
  cardiomyopathy, pericardial disease
  pericarditis
- Lung disease
  carcinoma of the bronchus; pulmonary embolus; pneumonia
- Metabolic
  thyrotoxicosis; alcohol abuse – acute and chronic
- Lone atrial fibrillation
  the term used to describe atrial fibrillation when no cause is discovered; this accounts for about 5% of cases.

3.29 Hypertension **Answers: A B D**

Hypertension may be essential (90%) or secondary (10%). This question refers to causes of secondary hypertension.

Renal causes include chronic glomerulonephritis and polycystic renal disease. Renal artery stenosis due to fibromuscular hyperplasia or atheroma may also cause hypertension. Renal causes are the most common cause of secondary hypertension.

Endocrine causes include Conn's syndrome, in which episodic muscular weakness occurs due to hypokalaemia. Other symptoms include tetany and nocturia. Phaeochromocytomas produce excess catecholamines that cause palpitations, tremor, sweating, headache, flushing, etc. Hypertension may be intermittent or constant and postural hypotension may be present (another common question). Tachycardia, bradycardia and other arrhythmias may occur. Flushing, fever and glycosuria are also features. Phaeochromocytoma may occur in association with other conditions, for example neurofibromatosis, Cushing's syndrome, acromegaly and hyperparathyroidism are also causes of secondary hypertension.

Cardiac causes include coarctation of the aorta. A systolic murmur near the midline of the back occurs.

Note that the question refers to the causes of hypertension and not the consequences which include retinal changes and ECG changes due to cardiac enlargement.

3.30 Jaundice **Answers: C D**

Dark urine in jaundice implies that there is an obstruction to conjugated bilirubin entering the bowel. This results in overspill of conjugated bilirubin into the urine producing a dark colour. Causes of obstructive jaundice include gallstones, biliary tract tumours, sclerosing cholangitis, and carcinoma of the head of the pancreas. These all cause extra-hepatic obstruction. Intra-hepatic biliary obstruction can occur with drugs such as nitrazepam.

When unconjugated bilirubin is in excess it is excreted into the urine. It has no colour, hence the term acholuric jaundice. Causes of this include:

- deficiency of conjugating enzymes, e.g. Gilbert's syndrome
- relative lack of functioning enzymes, e.g. infants who are breast-fed may develop physiological jaundice

3.58 Generalised lymphadenopathy **Answers: A C E**

See Paper 2, explanation 2.32. Other options that have been reported include rubella (true) and Still's disease (true).

3.59 Death certificates **Answers: B D E**

The important observations that need to be made before certifying death are:

- absence of response to external stimuli
- absence of a central pulse which must be felt for 1 minute
- absence of heart sounds for at least 1 minute
- absence of breath sounds for at least 1 minute
- both pupils must be non-reactive to light and must be fixed and dilated

The JVP is irrelevant and the radial pulse is not important as it is not a central pulse.

3.60 Angina **Answers: A B C D**

Angina may be precipitated by anaemia; this causes an increase in workload of the heart.

Thyroxine causes an increase in heart rate and cardiac output, and stress or emotion may provoke angina. Eating a large meal may increase the workload of the heart.

Myocardial infarction may actually cure angina. This is because ischaemia is painful but if that area dies due to infarction, it will no longer produce pain.

MCQ REVISION INDEX

The numbers after each entry refer to the examination and question number.

PASTEST BOOKS FOR MEDICAL STUDENTS

The Practical Guide to Medical Ethics and Law for Junior Doctors and Medical Students

M Brennan, C Baxter, Y Coldicott

- Excellent guidance on how to study ethics and law
- Practical guidance on how to pass your exams
- Real case studies from international doctors
- Top tips based on real life incidents

150 MCQs on Clinical Pharmacology and Therapeutics

D Hassanally & B Wasan

- 3 Practice Exams each containing 50 Multiple Choice Questions
- Detailed answers and expanded teaching notes
- A wide variety of MCQs presented in an easily accessible exam format

Clinical Skills for Medical Students: A Hands-on Guide

Bickle, Hamilton, et al

- Covers system-based chapter i.e. cardiovascular, respiratory with other common examinations
- Useful tips on how to write-up and present a case including case history
- Clear diagrams to explain difficult concepts

Radiology Casebook for Medical Students

R Wasan, A Grundy, R Beese

- Covers X-rays, MR and CT scans
- Read our guidance section to enhance your interpretation skills
- Take the test paper to confirm you are on the right track

EMQs for Medical Students Volumes 1 & 2

A Feather et al

Two volumes of EMQs covering all major themes. Written by doctors at the forefront of medical education with invaluable experience in writing best-sellers for medical students.

- Cover all topics likely to be assessed during medical training
- Over 100 themes contained in each volume
- Essential list of normal values

OSCEs for Medical Undergraduates Volumes 1 & 2
R Visvanathan, A Feather JSP Lumley
Volume 1 covers: Cardiovascular Diseases, Neurology, Psychiatry, Ophthalmology, Otolaryngology, Haematology, respiratory Medicine, Orthopaedics, Trauma, Ethics and Legal Medicine.
Volume 2 covers: Endocrinology, Gastroenterology, Urology, Renal Medicine, Obstetrics, Gynaecology, Rheumatology and Dermatology.
Each book covers:

- History taking, clinical examinations, investigations, practical techniques, making a diagnosis, prescribing treatment and other issues
- Answers and additional information so that you can assess your performance and identify areas needing further attention
- Contain X-rays, scans, haematological and biochemical results and a colour slide section

Surgical Finals: Passing the Clinical
Kuperberg & Lumley

- 90 examples of favourite long and short surgical cases
- Syllabus checklist for structured revision
- 18 detailed examination schemes with action tables
- 36 tables of differential diagnosis
- 134 popular viva questions for self-assessment
- Recommended reading list and revision index.

Medical Finals: Passing the Clinical
Moore & Richardson

- 101 typical long cases, short cases and spot diagnoses
- Syllabus checklist for systematic revision
- Vital tips on preparation and presentation
- Structured examination plans for all cases
- Concise teaching notes highlight areas most relevant to finals
- Revision index for easy access to specific topics

Surgical Finals: Structured Answer and Essay Questions
Visvanathan & Lumley

- Prepare for the written examination with this unique combination of essay questions and the new structured answer questions
- 111 structured answer questions with detailed teaching notes
- 52 typical essay questions with sample essay plans and model essays
- Invaluable revision checklist to help you to trach your progress
- Short textbook reviews enable you to select the best textbooks

Medical Finals: Structured Answer and Essay Questions
Feather, Visvanathan & Lumley

- Prepare for the written examination with this unique combination of essay questions and the new structured answer questions
- 141 structured answer questions with detailed teaching notes
- 73 typical essay questions with sample essay plans and model essays
- Invaluable revision checklist to help you to trach your progress
- Short textbook reviews enable you to select the best textbooks

150 Essential MCQs for Surgical Finals
Hassanally & Singh

- The crucial material for your exam success
- Extended teaching notes, bullet points and mnemonics
- Revision indexes for easy access to specific topics